Medical Tourism
and Inequity in India

The Anthropology of Tourism: Heritage, Mobility, and Society

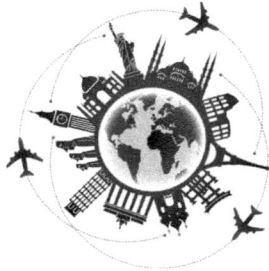

Series Editor: Michael A. Di Giovine
(West Chester University of Pennsylvania)

Mission Statement

The Anthropology of Tourism: Heritage, Mobility, and Society series provides anthropologists and others in the social sciences and humanities with cutting-edge and engaging research on the culture(s) of tourism. This series embraces anthropology's holistic and comprehensive approach to scholarship, and is sensitive to the complex diversity of human expression. Books in this series particularly examine tourism's relationship with cultural heritage and mobility and its impact on society. Contributions are transdisciplinary in nature, and either look at a particular country, region, or population, or take a more global approach. Including monographs and edited collections, this series is a valuable resource to scholars and students alike who are interested in the various manifestations of tourism and its role as the world's largest and fastest-growing source of socio-cultural and economic activity.

Advisory Board Members

Quetzil Castañeda, Saskia Cousin, Jackie Feldman, Nelson H. H. Graburn, Jafar Jafari, Tom Selwyn, Valene Smith, Amanda Stronza, Hazel Tucker, and Shinji Yamashita

Recent Titles in the Series

Medical Tourism and Inequity in India: The Hyper-Commodification of Healthcare by Kristen Smith

A Sacred Vertigo: Pilgrimage and Tourism in Rocamadour, France by Deana L. Weibel

Women and Tourist Work in Jamaica: Seven Miles of Sandy Beach by A. Lynn Bolles

Encounters across Difference: Tourism and Overcoming Subalternity in India by Natalia Bloch

Study Abroad and the Quest for an Anti-Tourism Experience edited by John Bodinger de Uriarte and Michael A. Di Giovine

Tourism and Language in Vieques: An Ethnography of the Post-Navy Period by Luis Galanes Valldejuli

The Ethnography of Tourism: Edward Bruner and Beyond edited by Naomi Leite, Quetzil E. Castañeda, and Kathleen M. Adams

Medical Tourism and Inequity in India

The Hyper-Commodification of Healthcare

Kristen Smith

LEXINGTON BOOKS
Lanham • Boulder • New York • London

Published by Lexington Books
An imprint of The Rowman & Littlefield Publishing Group, Inc.
4501 Forbes Boulevard, Suite 200, Lanham, Maryland 20706
www.rowman.com

86-90 Paul Street, London EC2A 4NE

British Library Cataloguing in Publication Information Available

Library of Congress Cataloging-in-Publication Data

Names: Smith, Kristen, 1976- author.
Title: Medical tourism and inequity in India : the hyper-commodification of healthcare / Kristen Smith.
Other titles: Anthropology of tourism: heritage, mobility, and society.
Description: Lanham, Maryland : Lexington Books, 2022. | Series: The anthropology of tourism : heritage, mobility, and society | Includes bibliographical references and index.
Identifiers: LCCN 2022001917 (print) | LCCN 2022001918 (ebook) | ISBN 9781793644176 (cloth) | ISBN 9781793644190 (paperback) | ISBN 9781793644183 (ebook)
Subjects: LCSH: Medical tourism—India. | Medical care—India.
Classification: LCC RA793.5 .S64 2022 (print) | LCC RA793.5 (ebook) | DDC 362.10954—dc23/eng/20220209
LC record available at https://lccn.loc.gov/2022001917
LC ebook record available at https://lccn.loc.gov/2022001918

For my amazing daughter Ajala.

Contents

List of Figures and Tables

FIGURES

TABLES

Acknowledgments

This book has been a long time in the making, and I am extremely grateful to the many people who have assisted and facilitated me in various ways. First, I would like to thank the members of my PhD Advisory committee for their intellectual guidance, support, and encouragement for the duration of my candidacy and beyond: Hans Baer, Richard Chenhall, Marcia Langton, and (earlier) Salim Lakha. I also want to thank all those in India who facilitated my fieldwork, sharing their experience, knowledge, kindness, and general support. First and foremost, I wish to extend my deepest gratitude to my mentor and chief informant in Mumbai, "Dr Nayar," for graciously welcoming me into the world of Mumbai hospitals, his family and home. Without his seemingly boundless generosity, this research would not have been possible. I also thank all those who participated in this research for their time, patience, shared knowledge and expertise.

I further acknowledge the Tata Institute for Social Sciences for hosting me during my fieldwork and the Centre for Health Equity, Melbourne School of Population and Global Health at The University of Melbourne, for providing funding for the research, office space, and other related resources during my PhD and beyond. For their varied help and guidance I thank all of my many colleagues over the past decade. I am particularly grateful for the support and encouragement of my colleagues at the Indigenous Studies Unit over the years.

During recent years, others have graciously offered me the privilege of their direct critical engagement with the materials and ideas for this book, particularly Polash Larson, Michael Di Giovine, and multiple other anonymous readers.

I also acknowledge and am grateful to the following institutions that provided funding for various elements of this research: the Faculty of

Arts, University of Melbourne; The Australian Government Department of Education, Employment and Workplace Relations (DEEWR) for the Endeavour Research Fellowship that enabled my fieldwork in Mumbai; and the Australian Association of Anthropology.

I thank my friends (in India and Australia) and family for their incredible patience, support, critical queries, and comments throughout this endeavor, notably Alana Gibson, my mother Judy and sister, Kellie. Also, a special thanks to my Hindi teacher and friend, Preethi, who welcomed me into her life and home, teaching me how to cook her favourite South Indian dishes and helping me navigate my way through day-to-day life in Mumbai. Thanks is also due to Mrs Gambhir, who helped me through many of the sometimes perplexing and usually entertaining episodes that unfolded during my time in Mumbai.

Last, but certainly not least, I acknowledge my incredible daughter Ajala for putting up with me as I dragged her across continents and threw her head-long into so many diverse and challenging situations from such a young age.

Introduction

Tensions, Conflicts, and Contradictions

The intensive privatization and commodification of healthcare across the globe has grown at an unprecedented rate over recent decades. Medical tourism has emerged within this context as an economic development strategy for many developing and emerging nations, and provisional remedy for patients facing escalating costs, long waiting periods, or lack of access to medical specialists at home. Yet, little is known about the complex and diverse implications of the growing industry for nations with developing or emerging economies, such as India. Similarly, we know little of the implications of the industry's fragility in the context of emergent global pandemics such as COVID-19 and the growing environmental and ecological crises: both disrupting the global travel required for the trade.

This book is based on a critical ethnographic study conducted in 2009–2010, following the footprint of medical tourism primarily across five large, private Trust hospitals in Mumbai, India, investigating the role of medical tourism in the local disruptions to the delivery of healthcare services, the healthcare workforce and the resident population. The ethnographic gaze was further dispersed across the greater city of Mumbai in consultancy rooms, cafes, university lecture halls, private homes, hotels, smaller not-for-profit hospitals, and a range of other spaces from rickshaw to boulevard. It was also entangled and engaged across less spatially definable locales, weaving its way across the transient domains of the Internet, media, and policy sphere.

The time I spent in India conducting fieldwork for this ethnography (2009–2010) coincided with a unique period of intensive commercial transition in the tertiary healthcare sector of India. Large private hospitals were constructed or in the midst of expansion across the city and nation, and many of the charitable Trust hospitals that had traditionally served the lower classes of the population were in the midst of major upgrades, while shifting to

1

corporate modes of operation and management. As with most contemporary ethnographic research, this research is grounded in local realities, but has significant global interconnections. The methodology used in the study created an analytical framework from which to examine local adverse impacts of the progressively commercialized practices and policy that have emerged in healthcare systems across the globe. A contextual and historical examination of structural economic, technological and health policy reform in India enabled a locally embedded investigation of the global shift away from inclusive social and public health approaches to market-led health models.

As such, this book explores the emerging life-worlds within globalizing tertiary biomedical institutions in Mumbai, and their role in the global healthcare service supply chain within intersecting religious, social, cultural, historical, and economic milieus, offering critical insights into the ever growing and dynamic complexities of the contemporary world. This microcosmic view of wider economic patterns of neoliberalism and commodification of goods and services transpiring within and between nations illustrates how healthcare services are rapidly transitioning from a human rights frame to that of merely another global commodity.

Much of the extant literature on medical tourism has focused on the plights and journeys of the medical tourists themselves, its economic and development prospects for different nations or the wide and varied legal implications of the trade. By contrast, this book focuses on the hosts of medical tourism: the tertiary healthcare institutions and healthcare workforce engaging in medical tourism and the local host population. In doing so, the book details how medical tourism is contributing to a transformation of understandings of health and healthcare for the professional workforce in India, the organizations they work within and the broader social, political, and economic structures of the nation. Using this transversal, processual approach, this book identifies the complex and dynamic links between medical tourism as a social phenomenon, and its particular connective processes, with consideration of the unfolding relations of power from within, and out, of the sites in which the research was situated.

One of the core propositions of this book is that medical tourism, as an industry and practice, is connected to local disruptions in the delivery of healthcare services to the resident population of Mumbai via the corporatization of institutions that deliver care, and its role in the hyper-commodification of the healthcare system at large. Further, it provides a view of the assemblages of transformational, territorial logics of power that the local Indian medical workforce operates within, of which medical tourism constitutes a key component.

The ethnographic research informing this book received research ethics approval from the University of Melbourne's Health Sciences Human Ethics

Sub-Committee. Across the book, pseudonyms are applied to all study informants and hospitals of focus to support the privacy and confidentiality of participants. For this reason, there are also no images of the individual hospitals of focus within in the book; however, several images of other Indian hospitals are used to provide a point of reference for the reader.

THE STUDY THROUGH THE LENS
OF THE ETHNOGRAPHER

I first visited Ramrakhyani Hospital[1] in mid-2009. It was one of the five, large, not-for-profit hospitals of focus for my ethnographic study of the life worlds of healthcare professionals in the context of medical tourism in the city. At the time, I had been living in Mumbai for three months, and had navigated my way via autorickshaw from my apartment in a far-eastern suburban neighborhood of Mumbai. Ramrakhyani was one of Mumbai's newest hospitals, built on the outskirts of the city. The building's grand architecture, palatial open planning, sky-high ceilings, and elegant, yet contemporary, décor externally signposted the class of patients, or "clientele" catered to within. As I made my way into the hospital, I approached the reception desk in the atrium and was greeted by a hospital "concierge" who directed me to a large, opulently adorned waiting area. At the time, I distinctly recall how fresh and cool the air was in comparison to the dusty-yet-damp, choking humidity outside that I had escaped from moments before.

The hospital was part of an exclusive, 250-acre estate made up of high-rise residential "society buildings," an international Cambridge International Examinations (CIE) school, a large business precinct, leisure center, five-star hotels, shopping mall, cinema, bars, restaurants, and its own railway station. The town planning of the area was distinctly different to the majority of Mumbai, with wide roads, meticulous landscaping, and neo-classical architecture. There were nearby swimming pools and clubhouses, a go-karting track, rock climbing facilities, and wide tracts of land dedicated to open gardens and public promenades. The streets were clean, wide, and paved. Trees and other greenery framed a central, crystal-clear, lake. In a somewhat controversial move, the developers had banned religious buildings within the township, to promote a more "cosmopolitan" lifestyle for residents. There were very few beggars on the streets and no visible sign of the slums that weave their way throughout the rest of the city.

Although situated on the outskirts of what is known as India's noisiest city, here there were no blasting horns from the myriad of vehicles choking other streets with traffic, no *masjids* blaring crackling calls to prayer through loudspeakers, no firecrackers cutting through the midday clamor. It was as if

I had located a calm oasis within the wider cacophony of the city. This place barely resembled the Mumbai with which I had started to become acquainted; it was a place of "other." This Mumbai—sanitized, modernized, high-tech, and upwardly mobile—is what many Indians would very much like the rest of the world to imagine when they think of their city and nation. It is a segment that houses wealthy expatriates from multinational organizations in upmarket condominiums, where Hollywood movies are screened as frequently as Bollywood movies, where money flows through the streets in abundance.

While sitting, waiting for a scheduled meeting with one of the younger hospital administrators, I could hear filtered snippets of a conversation between a man and a woman sitting only a few seats away. They were discussing a treatment plan for the surgery the woman was about to undergo. They had arrived in India only the day before from the United Kingdom and were anxiously waiting for their doctor to summon them into a consulting office. The consulting area was sparsely filled with well-dressed, well-groomed, middle- and upper-class Indians also waiting patiently to see their consultants. I was soon to discover that the Trust hospital had state-of-the-art medical equipment, a gymnasium, auditorium, air conditioning throughout, infection control protocols, and an attached nursing college with 189 nurses on staff.

Classified as a multispecialty teaching hospital, the institution offered 32 disciplines including renal, coronary, and liver transplants; bariatric; cancer; IVF and surrogacy; urogynecology; radiology; ear, nose, and throat (ENT); and ophthalmology. The hospital rooms varied from basic shared "economy" rooms to the "presidential suite," which was charged out at USD 450 per night, the equivalent of the best rooms offered at the five-star hotels located in the south of the city. The demand for the hospital's services had become evident in the short years since it had opened its doors; during this time, it had already expanded from a 130-bed to 240-bed hospital. The hospital was managed by the philanthropic branch of a well-known property developer group in India, best known for creating nine separate townships on the outskirts of the Greater City of Mumbai. The two brothers who co-founded the property development group had recently featured in the "top 100 richest" list of Forbes Magazine.

In the year prior to my arrival in Mumbai, the Indian–Australian author Aravind Adiga won the esteemed United Kingdom Booker Prize for his novel "The White Tiger" (Adiga 2008). It is a ferocious, first person narrative from the perspective of a disaffected young man attempting to claw his way out of poverty and servitude, and the calculated, yet indifferent malevolence he employs to do so. Through a modified version of the Hegelian master–slave dialectic, the novel brings to life a tale of two Indias: the privileged, entitled India of the "haves" and the brutal, dehumanizing India of the "have-nots." It is a tale of the powerful and the powerless.

Despite Ramrakhyani's not-for-profit status, it was firmly connected to the India of the "haves." All the same, it stood a mere 45-minute autorickshaw commute from my apartment in the suburb of Govandi, an area of "have-nots." Govandi is home to Mumbai's largest abattoir, manifold slums (both legal and illegal), over 600 tenements, and the highest rates of tuberculosis and infant mortality in the city. The area's largest slum, Shivaji Nagar, is a resettlement colony of 300,000 people, densely crowded into a 1.3-square-kilometer area. It is home to thousands of migrants that flock to Mumbai every year from across the nation (Mili 2011, 82). The walls and uneven pavements of Govandi are awash with the red stains of *paan* spittle that need to be dodged on a regular basis as it sprays from buses, motorcycles, autorickshaws, and taxis lurching their way in and out of the narrow crevices utilized as streets. The smoke from human remains burned at the open-air crematorium 100 meters from my apartment regularly snaked through the dripping humidity to join forces with the city's acrid smog.

Large black kites—known as *shite-hawks* in British military slang—circled the area in flocks like vultures, riding the thermal currents and diving down to scavenge whatever live prey and carrion they could locate within the debris. Rats, the size of rabbits scuttled in and out of residential homes, *jhopadpattis*, street markets, and restaurants. It has been reported that the vast majority of the city's estimated 88 million rats are located in Govandi and the nearby slum of Dharavi (Buncombe 2012). Merely a stone's throw away, thousands of rag pickers—mainly women and children—eke out a daily living by filtering through and reselling anything of value they find in the vast toxic waste

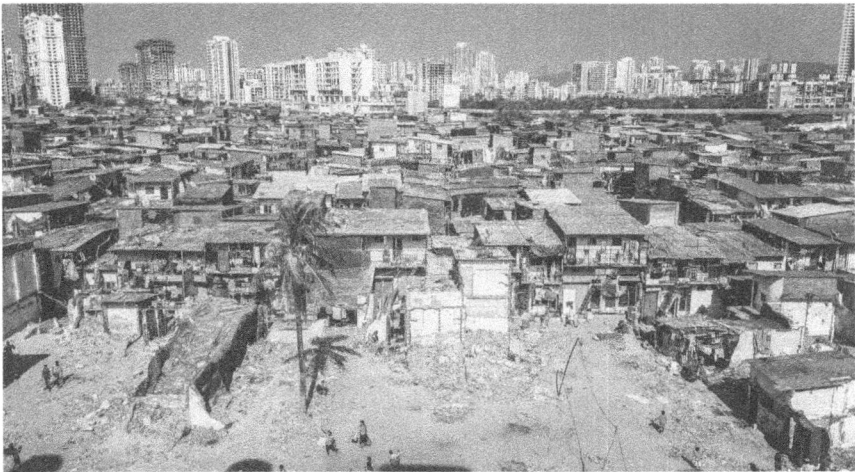

Figure 0.1   Aerial View of a Jhopadpatti in North-east Mumbai. *Source*: Ameeq (2020). Architecture/Buildings. Pixabay.

of the 130-hectare Deonar dumping ground, also reputedly one of the largest in Asia. This book and the research on which it draws is set in the midst of these two Indias, and inescapably, within the wider international milieu of the world's "haves" and "have-nots."

THE GLOBAL TRADE OF MEDICAL TOURISM

During the first two decades of the 21st century, promotional material originating from industry and the governments alike suggested that the dynamic growth of the medical tourism industry was set to explode internationally. Reports on the global economic status of this service industry were wide-ranging and often industry based, but the aggressive development of medical tourism in countries such as India, Thailand, and Malaysia indicated the importance that was placed on the sector as a vehicle for future economic development. From international trade agreements to national- and state-level policies, the economic impetus for emerging and developing nations with the capacity to attract international medical tourists was evident.

India positioned itself as one of the front-runners in the global medical tourism market, forging a reputation for their delivery of "value" tertiary healthcare services such as cardiac, cosmetic, and joint surgery. Hospitals, medical travel companies, private practices, and other third-party agents offered packages that included medical services, accommodation, air travel, bookings, and the arrangement of tourist retreats and tours for the recuperation period.

Although distinctive new trends and patterns emerged during this time, international travel for health and wellness has an extensive history. From as early as the Neolithic period, people traveled long distances to specific geographic locations across Europe to engage in health-related activities. These practices continued in varying forms throughout medieval times and by the 18th century, the upper strata of European classes regularly traveled across borders to bathe in thermal springs for perceived medical purposes. India, in particular, has an extensive and sacred history of pilgrimage, hospitality, death, and healing that is dynamically interwoven with the structures, processes, and promotion of medical tourism.

Although health-related travel is not a new phenomenon, the global direction of patient travel has gradually shifted away from individuals travelling from poorer countries to richer destination countries to access health services unavailable at home, to that of individuals from richer countries travelling to poorer nations (Connell 2011; Ormond 2014). Since the Asian financial crises of the late nineties, more affluent citizens from Asian countries who had previously traveled to the United States or Singapore for healthcare services no longer had the economic capacity to do so.

It was at this time that Bumrungrad Hospital in Thailand began to attract many international patients, becoming one of the most well-known medical tourist destinations in the world. This trend intensified after the September 11 attacks in New York, discouraging Arab citizens from travelling to the United States for healthcare. Between 2001 and 2006, the number of Arab citizens treated at Bumrungrad rose from 5,000 to 93,000 (de Arellano 2007). Bumrungrad Hospital also recorded shifts in the types of healthcare services sought by international patients, with the high ratio of cosmetic surgery reducing in favor of noncosmetic procedures. By 2007, noncosmetic treatments made up approximately 80% of treatments received by Americans at Bumrungrad (MacReady 2007). Milstein and Smith (2006) argued that this was a direct consequence of the struggling healthcare system in the United States, where a marked increase in insurance premiums, coupled with the growth of out-of-pocket payments left many of the populace unable to access affordable healthcare at home.

This "new" niche market of medical tourism emerged across and within developed and developing countries. The motivations of patients varied but were primarily related to real or imagined inadequacies of healthcare provision in countries of residence. Considerations included affordability of treatment; quality of services; duration of treatment waiting periods; and availability of specific treatments.

Cuba was one of the first countries to actively promote this new form of medical tourism. From the early 1960s, the Cuban government embarked on a program of medical internationalism, sending Cuban medical professionals to assist in mainly Latin American and African nations, and bringing international medical students and patients (medical tourists) back to Cuba for treatment. In the early 1990s, the Cuban government advertised "sun and surgery" packages including dental, cardiac, organ transplant, and cosmetic procedures in conjunction with spa or "wellness adventures." It has been estimated that over the course of 1995–1996, 25,000 medical tourists spent approximately USD 25 million on health-related treatments in the nation (de Arellano 2014, 292).

Goodrich and Goodrich (1987, 217) conducted one of the earliest scholarly studies of medical tourism, developing an initial definition of the term as "the attempt on the part of a tourist facility (e.g., hotel) or destination (e.g., Baden, Switzerland) to attract tourists by deliberately promoting its healthcare facilities, in addition to its regular tourist amenities." Goodrich (1993) later noted that the terms used by those studying the phenomena from a marketing perspective have shifted their terminology from medical tourism to healthcare tourism, to health tourism, respectively. In subsequent years, all three labels have been used broadly and somewhat interchangeably, with other recent additions such as medical value travel and medical outsourcing.

Despite medical tourism remaining the most commonly used, the range and inconsistency of the terminology applied in the broader literature to describe this sector indicates the lack of definitional consensus within the academe and beyond. An early attempt to delineate different forms of international health-seeking behavior, Henderson (2004) divided healthcare tourism into the three categories of medical tourism, cosmetic surgery tourism, and spas and alternative therapies tourism. However, Henderson's rationale of these categories highlights numerous preconceptions regarding different forms of health services. For example, Henderson describes cosmetic surgery as "non-essential treatments," and spa and alternative therapies as "hedonistic" pursuits, implying that medical tourism, conversely, describes essential treatments. Such dichotomies also serve to support and reinforce notions of the hierarchical dominance of biomedicine over and above the plurality of medical systems (indigenous, complementary, and alternative) internationally.

In contrast to Henderson's definition, Connell (2011, 11) has suggested that "medical tourism" serves as an umbrella term, "where and when patients travel overseas often over considerable distances, to take advantage of medical treatments which are not available or easily accessible (in terms of costs and waiting time) at home." Connell emphasizes here that medical tourism is primarily a response to inadequate healthcare systems in the home countries of patients. Importantly, Connell's definition, unlike most, incorporates the industry, collective and individual practice. In this book, I refer to medical tourism similarly, as a global, service-based industry, of which the practice can be viewed from both collective and individual perspectives. Although medical tourism of any form can occur within and across nations, this book focuses on international medical tourism and the impact and interactions of this industry with social actors and groups within nations promoting this service.

When entering the term "medical tourism" into an online search engine, it returns over 700 million hits, with hospitals, medical travel agencies, government and other agencies from all over the world providing tips, medical tourism packages, warnings and economic projections of the trade. There are emerging international hubs of expertise in niche health and wellness areas across the globe. For example, Thailand is widely considered the international leader in sex-reassignment surgery. The *Bloomberg Business* reported that at least 100 surgeons in Thailand are qualified to perform these surgeries, with their predominant business emerging from foreign patients (Gale 2015).

Luxury Cruise Ship medical tourism is another form of medical tourism projected to grow, where "floating hospitals" staffed by medical professionals transport intended "consumers" to international waters, potentially offering procedures that circumvent specific local regulations. For example, in 2021, amidst the emerging global Covid-19 pandemic, the Alaskan government advertised "vaccination cruises," offering free coronavirus vaccinations to encourage tourism within the nation. Although this variation of medical tourism has not yet developed beyond individual cruises offering "wellness and cruise" packages as a one of a wider array of offerings, it is but one of many new configurations of healthcare service delivery operating under the umbrella term of "medical tourism."

Despite the growing rates of medical tourism internationally, there remains very little empirical knowledge about the volume, nature, and broader practices of the multiple forms of medical tourism. Further, dominant discourses emerging from stakeholders such as policy makers, healthcare practitioners, governments, industry, and other related bodies are firmly situated within an economic frame. In this book, I describe both the short- and long-term implications of medical tourism for destination countries and patient origin nations, paying particular attention to the potential risks and harms it produces, particularly for vulnerable and marginalized groups within developing countries.

Much of the anthropological and other social science research conducted on medical tourism has been directed toward the hopes, motivations, and experiences of patients, or the types and forms of expectations of the national destinations attracting and hosting the healthcare consumers. By contrast, there has been far less scholarly attention examining the local effects of the growing phenomenon on the places, populations, industries, social structures, and healthcare systems in the local areas the services are provided. In this book, I focus on the local institutions and stakeholders engaging in the phenomenon, examining the underlying structural causes that drive patients to undertake medical treatment away from their place of residence. Although there has been much economic, physical, and symbolic investment from public and private institutions, there has been little interrogation of the dominant notions circulated globally that medical tourism will provide positive outcomes for host nations by driving economic development and, who the predominant beneficiaries of the industry and the practice are at any given time and place.

FOLLOWING THE FOOTPRINTS
OF MEDICAL TOURISM

Conceptualizing the research design for this study emerged over the course of several years. I was primarily interested in the systemic and structural impact of medical tourism on the large number of people within India who continue to live in dire poverty, aware that in all likelihood, any links between the two would be indirect and fraught with social and political sensitivities. However, the possibility of locating the research within one of

Mumbai's *jhopadpattis*, was unlikely to enable access to the broader power structures related to medical tourism that I was interested in. To investigate the impact of medical tourism on the "powerless," the next step was to embed the research in the culture of the "powerful" in the elite medical setting of large, private hospitals.

Establishing and maintaining contacts is the key to all ethnographic fieldwork, both to gain entrée to the site and to attain any other necessary permission that may be needed for the study to proceed. In this case, prior to commencing the research, a variety of official authorizations were required, including a university affiliation and access to a local academic supervisor to access a research visa. Further, and most importantly, I had to determine how to gain, navigate, and maintain access to the hospitals. In the context of the ongoing privatization of tertiary healthcare internationally, this was not a straightforward nor easy task. Inhorn (2004), discusses some of the methodological challenges represented by medical privatization within the context of her IVF research in the Middle East. She notes that to undertake hospital ethnographies, particularly in developing nations, the "ethnographer must gain access to private hospital spaces, which requires finding a medical "patron" who will allow this" (p. 2096). As fieldwork progressed, I grew more appreciative of the value of the association with the Tata Institute of Social Sciences (TISS) and their chosen mentor, Dr Nayar. Without the auspicing of my work under TISS and my mentor, this research would not have been possible.

In one of the first meetings I had with my key informant and patron at his hospital in South Mumbai, he gathered together a group of whom he affectionately called his "bosses." They were the next in the line of command at the hospital, the heads of departments. We started with a general discussion about the state of medical tourism and healthcare more broadly in India. The discussion soon shifted to what they thought was the best way for me, as a researcher, to capture and understand the broader picture of medical tourism in the country. Dr Nayar, at this point, turned to me and mentioned that I should keep in mind the story of the elephant and blind men when trying to understand the medical tourism industry in India. This is an Indian parable, which crosses religious, and caste lines, and also can be used to capture some of the difficulties and challenges of research design. The parable tells the tale of several blind men who come across an elephant for the first time. They are not told what is before them but are asked to examine the creature and describe it. The men begin to touch the body of the elephant. One man, after feeling the elephant's leg exclaims that it is like a pillar. Another man touches the elephant's trunk and describes the elephant as like a tree branch. The story continues with each man describing the elephant differently depending upon which section of the elephant they touched.

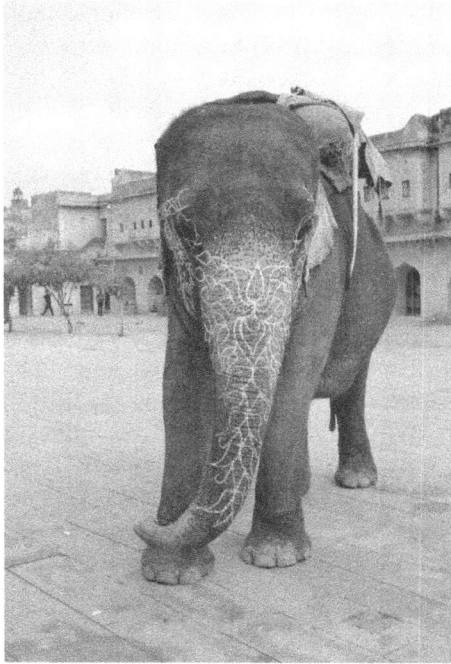

Figure 0.2   The Elephant and the Blind Ethnographer. *Source*: Ameeq (2020). Yolanda Coervers. Animals. Pixabay.

Dr Nayar finally explained, to the delighted chuckles of his staff, that this fable should warn me of the dangers of relying on any one perspective offered by the people I was researching, including himself. I was the one and only blind (wo)man, he reasoned, and although I would come across different viewpoints and contradictory conclusions, all would distinctly and uniquely form parts of one and the same elephant. A slight transposition of this allegory reveals one of the advantages of what was to become a multisited hospital ethnography of medical tourism. If medical tourism was the metaphorical elephant, and I was interested in the elephant itself, and its impact on its surrounds, then following its tracks and investigating the multiple sites and situations in which the elephant was embedded would enable in-depth understandings of how the elephant is located within a complex and dynamic web of local and global associations, connections, and relationships.

Thus, my field spanned the five hospitals in Mumbai, but also included the wider metropolis and beyond, entangled and engaged across less spatially and temporally definable settings, or scapes; the "onlife" and online transient domains of the Internet, media, and policy sphere. During my fieldwork, I spent varying periods conducting interviews and participant observation in the hospitals across the city. I examined multiple facets of the hospitals, including the broader policy structures, administrative functions, and the interactions, or what Del Vecchio Good (1995) describes as "clinical narratives," across wards and consultancy rooms. Ethnographic techniques allowed for an insight into the understandings and behaviors of the people I studied, facilitating a "glimpse behind the public masks and front-stage performances of social actors to backstage and often hidden arena of experience and social interaction" (Singer and Baer 2012, 59).

Ethnographies undertaken primarily within hospitals generally allow the researcher to act as a participant in the setting in one of three roles: the professional, the patient, or the visitor. Many anthropologists, particularly when researching the professional's point of view, have occupied the role of a medical professional. However, having no medical training, no medical ailments requiring treatment, and very little disciplinary empathy from my gatekeepers, my role in the hospitals was generally relegated to that of the visitor, an observing participant rather than the participant observer.

I observed the day-to-day interactions between a wide spectrum of health professionals, patients and their families, hospital management, and other financial and administrative staff. This approach had its limitations, I engaged myself in the activities on specific wards, attended administrative and management meetings, and generally "hung about" in these clinical settings over the course of a year. This phase of data collection occurred across the entire span of the fieldwork, however, the intensity was highly sporadic and required constant (re)negotiation of access to the field sites. Although management of all five hospitals had provided approval to conduct my fieldwork, what this meant and the way it was understood and interpreted by myself and those granting access fluctuated rapidly, sometimes on a daily basis.

Most of the gatekeepers in the hospitals tolerated but did not particularly appreciate the utility of my lengthy observations. Despite explanations, most maintained that they themselves could tell me all I needed to know without further "wasting" my time. Many of the senior administrators involved in the study maintained that I should busy myself with far more "useful" activities, such as conducting wide-scale surveys to capture what they saw as the more valuable and beneficial quantitative data. Given this general perception, it was fortuitous that the hospitals were very busy places, with healthcare staff working long and frenetic hours, lending itself to the need for spending many hours in the hospitals waiting for interviews and meetings to transpire, striking up conversations with the wide array of people wandering in and around the hospitals.

Although I spent considerable time in the hospitals, most of my fieldwork was spent doing what Forsythe (1999) calls the "invisible work" of ethnographic practice around and across the wider city in a variety of activities, both formal and informal. This was undertaken from the perspective of my multiple roles as: a member of the academic research community; "expatriate" in a large, business-driven city with a (relatively) small population of international residents; employer of household domestic staff; and mother of a primary-school-aged child, who attended a local school in Chembur. This invisible work included meeting with informants, undertaking archival research in media archives and lecturing and engaging with hospital administration students at TISS. I spent significant periods of time in local neighborhoods chatting with *chai-wallahs*, visiting acquaintances in the *jhopadpattis*, exploring the city's libraries, and visiting local hospitals and clinics. I participated in local festivals, attended social events, navigated the public transport system, trawled through the bazaars, and visited many temples and *masjids*. At one stage, my daughter and I even spent several days on set as extras in a Bollywood television serial. During fieldwork, I also traveled across multiple other states in India and other regions within Maharashtra.

As with many ethnographies, this study uses a complementary array of epistemological frameworks, research methods, and writing techniques. One such is what Kohn (2010) labels "mobile reflexivity," where the researcher views herself as an ethnographic resource (rather than abstracted neutral observer/analyst). In this form of reflexivity, both serendipity and memory play a significant and complex role in the production of the text (Kohn 2010). Mobile reflexivity attends to the dynamic repositioning in the construction of meaning that is undertaken by a researcher as a social actor, accounting for movements across both time and space. Specific narrative techniques I use in this book include the reconstruction of self-narratives of serendipity in the field from my more "visceral memories," where I make my "self" explicitly visible in the ethnography. This literary approach aims to address some of the tensions between the subjective and objective representations within the ethnography by highlighting the voices of my informants as well as my engagement with them.

THE EMERGENCE OF MEDICAL TOURISM IN A HYPERCOMMODIFIED HEALTHCARE SYSTEM

This book examines the period of transition in India during which hospitals were engaged in a process of intense commercialization of medical care (late 2000s and early 2010s), in the context of the hyper-commodification of healthcare across the nation. The book is situated in this liminal and transitional period, employing ethnographic descriptions augmented with data drawn from international and national datasets and archival sources to critically unpack and explore the impact of relevant policy and politics in India and beyond. As such, it provides insight into an uneven, and often highly undocumented process.

In chapters 1 and 2, I introduce and contextualize the ethnography, deconstructing some of the relevant nomenclature of medical tourism, the structure of the industry, and some of the central themes explored within the book. Chapter 1 outlines the book's theoretical engagement with critical medical anthropology and rights-based approaches, within an overarching social justice frame. It also looks at the mounting ideological frictions emerging with the growth of medical tourism, and how the nomenclature itself points to the paradoxes evident in the industry and practice. Competing understandings of health as a basic right or a commodity are at the heart of this paradox, whereby the coalescence of health within a commercial tourism frame fortifies the global ideological turn toward health as a commodity.

In chapter 2, the national and global theoretical (and demographic) context of the book is presented, detailing some of the key debates pertaining to globalization, economic development, and consumerism in the context of the biopolitics of medical tourism. The chapter outlines the role of international institutions in the hyper-commodification of the Indian healthcare system, with a particular focus on the introduction of structural adjustment macroeconomic programs and policies within the nation. In doing so, the chapter outlines some of the historical processes and conditions that led to biomedicine's economic dominance over Ayurveda, Yoga and Naturopathy, Unani, Siddha, and Homeopathy (AYUSH) systems in India. Drawing on data from international and national sources, the macro context of Indian health and healthcare within which medical tourism is embedded is presented, comparing and contrasting key population health and demographic indicators in India to other nations promoting medical tourism services. These data indicate that although there has been some improvement in India's population health in recent decades, many critical issues remain. In particular, the inequitable distribution of health outcomes, healthcare funding, access, infrastructure and human resources has widened exponentially over past decades.

In chapter 3, the significance of "tourism" within the phenomenon of medical tourism is described, with a focus how hospital practices were transforming, replicating those of the (nonmedical) tourism industry. The chapter describes the rise of international tourism more broadly in India, and its increasing function within the national economy. The agency of different actors engaging in medical tourism are also described, from the local private Trust hospitals in the study, through to international stakeholders, such as multilateral institutions and multinational corporations. This chapter explores medical tourism branding as a form of affective work, arising from the hospitals, healthcare workforce, government, and other third-party stakeholders. It also looks at how different marketing tactics used in the hospitals correspond with and relate to tourism, supporting and reinforcing notions of market-led healthcare. The impact of multiscaled disruptive "events" on medical tourism is examined, including global pandemics, in alignment with wider practices of tourism.

In chapter 4, the focus shifts to a core dilemma illuminated by this study, exploring local manifestations of the impact of the commodification of healthcare on tertiary healthcare institutions in India, with particular attention paid to disruptions in the not-for-profit sector. The history and religious traditions related to philanthropy in India are also outlined, contextualizing the role this sector has played in servicing the underserved population. Detailed histories of several Trust hospitals in the study illustrate how shifting forms of governance and management from religious or philanthropic to corporate, have transformed the sector, particularly with regard to escalating costs of out-of-pocket treatments. The Trust hospitals of the nation have serviced a considerable proportion of the Indian population from early colonization, particularly the vulnerable and marginalized. Thus, these corporate transformations pose significant challenges for the healthcare system, placing an unsustainable upward pressure on the extremely under resourced public tertiary healthcare sector.

Chapter 5 focuses on the local engagement of healthcare professionals with discourses of neoliberal development and the transformational, territorial logics of power of which medical tourism constitutes a key component. The chapter traces the structural context, professional perceptions, aspirations, and day-to-day activities in the lives of healthcare professionals working in private hospitals within the city of Mumbai. A comparison of the management and operational workings within different hospitals, the staff configurations, and the shifting modes of power (both symbolically and structurally) explores the working conditions experienced by physicians and other health workers in the tertiary institutions of India. This context provides a base from which to better understand of the role, function, and effect of medical tourism on healthcare workers in India. Several ethnographic examples further outline the impact of medical tourism on professional practice, such as how the imaginaries of the expectations of a "global patient" are translated by health professionals and embedded in their work.

Chapter 6 addresses the particular set of systemic, systematic, and sociospatial practices and functions that are indirectly, yet intimately, connected to the emergence and growth of medical tourism, and associated health inequities in India. Drawing on critiques of the commodification of healthcare, the chapter details how and why the tertiary healthcare sector has become a site of exclusion for the population's "have-nots" and an enclave of exclusivity for the "haves" (both within the nation and for medical tourists across the globe). This form of zoning is not exclusive to the healthcare sector. It is replicated in many forms across the city of Mumbai, with "gated islands" dotting the landscape, affording entry to only the privileged of the populace. The emergence of these sociospatial microcosms of exclusivity is indicative of the structural economic patterns of inequity rapidly escalating across the city and the nation.

Drawing on earlier chapters, the final chapter examines how medical tourism is understood, practiced, and regulated in India in the context of the hyper-commodification of healthcare in local and global contexts. Here, I argue that medical tourism has failed to deliver on the benevolent rhetoric that it facilitates access to health services for "all." Rather, it is segmented and directed toward specific social and economic substructures and international subpopulations. Focusing on the local nuanced effects at the sites of medical tourism and addressing the contribution of medical tourism to the widening health equity gap in Mumbai, this chapter synthesizes how the book builds on our knowledge of the intersections between local and international circuits of power, the political economy of healthcare systems, and the structures and substructures that impact on the delivery of health services to human populations.

The widening "cracks" in India's healthcare system detailed across this book reveal the high vulnerability of the nation's population to public health crises, as demonstrated by the emergence of the COVID-19 pandemic. New, more virulent variants of the virus emerged in early 2021, leading to escalating rates of infection, morbidity, and mortality across the country. This highlighted the critical deficiencies of the national healthcare system, particularly in the public sector. The under-resourcing and consequent shortages within the health workforce, medical supplies, equipment, and hospital beds were starkly revealed to a global audience, as national daily infections peaked at over 400,000 new cases per day in May 2021. The inability of India's healthcare system to attenuate the experience of the pandemic by providing the localized or nationwide public health response required to protect or treat its citizens during this crisis underscores the failure of the neoliberal pro-privatization policies established in the healthcare system in the early 1990s.

It is within this hypercommodified, intensively privatized context that medical tourism has flourished in India over the past two decades, yet to what end and for whom? And importantly, how does the industry impact on the hosts and host population of medical tourism destinations? These core questions are addressed across this book within a social justice and rights-based frame, seeking to disrupt, deconstruct, and reconceptualize perspectives of medical tourism in India, and globally.

NOTE

1. I have used pseudonyms throughout this book for all of my informants.

Chapter 1

"First World Treatment at Third World Prices"

STUDYING UP: A CRITICAL, RIGHTS-BASED APPROACH

This book draws on political economy approaches from critical medical anthropology (CMA) and rights-based approaches (RBAs) in a critique of medical tourism that explicitly challenges the reductive dualisms (e.g., empowered or disempowered health seeker vs empowered or disempowered host nation/provider) emerging from dominant discourses. It does so by addressing the circuits of medical tourism production and consumption, and engaging with issues of power, equity, and development processes. The agency, or lack thereof, of the health seeker is often the focus of many anthropologists studying medical tourism, with the structural and material inequalities generated by the medical tourism industry, economy and workplace often absent or relegated as a minor consideration.

Over three decades ago, Laura Nader (1969) first challenged anthropologists to take a "vertical slice" through both systems and institutions to analyze cultures of the powerful and the ways in which they operate, casting the ethnographic gaze on the institutions at the core of capitalist processes. Although medical anthropologists predominantly engaged in applied theory and practice up until the early 1980s, a subfield emerged using a political economy approach, drawing heavily on Wallerstein's (1974a, 1974b, 1979) world systems theories and Frank's (1969, 1978, 1984) version of dependency theory. This subfield, CMA, called for a move beyond benevolent understandings of economic and political policies (Singer and Baer 1995), with the view that "health ideas and practices reinforce social inequality as well as expressing it" (Sobo 2011, 18). Most CMA approaches focus on the vertical links between the local groups and context studied and the "larger regional, national, and global human society" (Singer and Baer 2012, 39). This multilevel analysis incorporates the macro-social, meso-social, and micro-social in relation to the operation of health systems, placing all social institutions and actors within this frame of reference. It is through this frame that CMA investigates imbalances of power and domination that operate across and within local, regional, national, and international settings. Particular attention is paid to distribution, which affects the way that sickness and healing is considered and acted upon (Singer and Baer 2012).

CMA also views biomedicine as one of many ethno-medicines, albeit the predominant form in contemporary societies. CMA challenges the reductionist approach of orthodox medical anthropology, shifting the analytical gaze to the largely ignored ideological features of biomedicine. These include the conceptual support that the natural sciences bring to notions of medical control over human beings and the contribution of medical science in (re) production patterns of dominance through esoteric scientific knowledge and standards of excellence. CMA approaches posit that biomedicine's hierarchical dominance in the international system is a result of the emergence of industrial capitalism, which was elevated due to its ideological compatibility with the growth of the international market economy and through its capacity to support the dominant capitalist class (Waitzkin 2000). Further, CMA centralizes the role of social aspects of health, attending to local issues within macro power structures, processes, and relations. Theoretical concepts, including that of biopower and structural violence, have been usefully applied to complex global and local public health issues to reconceptualize perspectives of the social forces underlying our understandings of health and illness more broadly.

Similarly to CMA, fields of development studies and human rights scholarship evolved in the 1990s into a broad, and arguably radical, theoretical platform: an RBA to development theory (Anand and Sen 2000; Farmer 1999; Nussbaum 1997; Sen and Dreze 1999). Prior to this time, human rights theory and practice centered on civil and political rights within specific legal frameworks. The union between the two fields emerged from debates calling both perspectives into question: development theories for their neoliberal bias and RBAs for their epistemological grounding in Western Enlightenment ideology. In response, a general appeal for rights to incorporate broader social justice conceptualizations arose, usually framed within economic, social, and cultural rights, emphasizing principles of equality for all (Mohan and Holland 2001). The view of health as a human right has evolved alongside other human rights discourses. The influential 1978 Alma Ata Conference and consequent Declaration expressly states that health is a human right, requiring engagement with a wide range of other social and economic configurations to realize maximal health.

From an RBA, individuals are viewed as active agents of change, in contrast to simply beneficiaries of rights. RBAs identify accountability by outlining the responsibilities and duties of states to ensure rights are upheld. RBAs also refer to a wide range of human rights, generally falling under the common categories of participation and empowerment, good governance, social and economic rights. An RBA encourages participation in the politicization of social and economic rights, enhancing the position of people, or groups, as active rights holders and creators, rather than passive agents. RBAs also attempt to create systemic change through the application of rights across all stages of development, interrogating and challenging when needed, embedded assumptions situated in prevailing ideologies. Thus, an RBA calls into question the moral and ethical underpinnings of market-led healthcare and healthcare systems, examining global shifts toward the commodification of healthcare and consequent mounting frictions between the competing principles of healthcare as a commodity or a right.

ENCOUNTERS OF "TOURISM" IN MEDICAL TOURISM

The appropriateness of the term "medical tourism" is widely debated in the scholarly literature, with many criticizing its use for "its inability, at best, to capture the desperation felt by patients crossing borders for medical care and for its ability, at worst, to undermine the formal and informal recognition by others of that desperation" (Ormond and Lunt 2020, 4183). Bochaton and Lefebvre (2009) have argued opposition to the term are related to the contradictions raised by the coupling of "leisure and pleasure with disease, suffering and treatment," and the consequent links inferred between consumerism and healthcare (2009, 98). Some medical tourists have also publicly expressed their indignation toward the term. For example, the partner of a citizen from the United States who traveled to India for heart surgery due to a lack of health insurance coverage in the United States commented at a hearing before the United States Congress, "we were not tourists seeking an inexpensive, exotic vacation while having medical treatment. We were fighting for Howard's life" (*The Globalization of Healthcare: Can Medical Tourism Reduce Healthcare Costs?* 2006). The contention here, again, is that the label "tourism" evokes a light-heartedness and level of triviality to life that disregards the trauma involved in engaging in this form of activity. If a patient is driven to seek treatment overseas by economic or socio-political forces, it is perceived as inappropriate to link tourism to the practice.

Similarly, some medical anthropologists have rejected the label medical tourism, using instead the term "medical travel" (Kangas 2002, 2010; Smith-Morris and Manderson 2010; Song 2010; Whitakker and Spier 2010).

Whittaker and Spier (2010), for example, have stressed the need for more "appropriate neutral definitions" due to the range of people undertaking this type of activity and the "intimations of hedonism" the term "tourism" implies (Whittaker and Speier 2010a: 370). Others have instead rejected the term arguing that medical tourism does not sufficiently politicize the phenomena, asserting terms such as "medical exile" or "biomedical pilgrimage" would more effectively capture the medical marginalization of patients traveling internationally to seek healthcare (Milstein and Smith 2006; Inhorn and Patrizio 2009; Song 2010; Ormond and Kaspar 2018).

However, in both scholarly and mainstream debates of medical tourism, scanty few have engaged with the vast body of work and theorization that has developed in contemporary critical tourism studies. Connell (2013) too has questioned this lack of engagement with "tourism" beyond that of nomen-clature in the international medical tourism literature. Notable exceptions include the edited book in this series, *Tourism and Wellness: Travel for the Good of All?* edited by Grimwood and others (2018), Connell's (2011, 2013, 2015) work on medical tourism, and Bochaton and Lefebvre's (2009) excel-lent chapter "The rebirth of the hospital: Heterotopia and medical tourism in Asia" in *Asia on Tour*.

The perception of tourism as a flippant practice is based on an outdated, essentialist "idea of the tourist solidified as an all-encompassing analytical monolith" (Winter, Teo, and Chang 2009, 4–5), of which contemporary studies of tourism have moved beyond. Rather, critical studies of tourism are placed within broader social, cultural, political, and economic contexts, addressing a wide range of issues including "aesthetics, postcolonialism, heritage, healthcare and nation-building" (Winter et al. 2009, 6). These approaches attend to both the individual practice and the wider emerging pat-terns related to the collective.

In the context of the varied experiences, practices and patterns of tourism, differentiated experiences, motivations and practices of individual tourists do not preclude, as claimed, that its consumption is structured by "the material inequalities of wealth and opportunity, which are differentiated according to class, ethnicity, gender and sexuality" (Bianchi 2009, 488). Although a medi-cal tourist may experience structural inequities at home preventing access to local medical treatment, their global socioeconomic status still facilitates transnational access to high-quality care in other nations such as India. This is regardless of whether the transnational mobility is north–south, south–north, intra-north, or intra-south. However, if much of the Indian population is unable to access healthcare at home for similar reasons, there are no such options or choices from which to seek cross-border care. Many people across the globe similarly do not have the economic capacity to seek care beyond their own borders. What this highlights is that medical tourism is an outward representation of the inequities operating in local and international markets. It is also a driving force that acts to reinforce and reproduce these inequities (see chapter 6 for more detail).

Deconstructing these discourses of the nomenclature medical tourism highlights the significance of the tourism encountered in medical tourism. The benefit of a tourism frame for this book is that it trains the ethnographic gaze to the processes of commodification that are central to the growth of the industry and collective global practice. If we accept medical tourism as a service-based commodity, then we must also recognize that its symbolic properties are shaped at the interface of health consumer desires, industry marketing and the differentiated experiences, motivations and practices of individuals, and the collective. Importantly, it unveils the global material inequalities premising the industry, regardless of the experience of any individual medical tourist. Medical tourism is a driving force that acts to reinforce and reproduce inequities, signaling that some people (i.e., the global middle-classes and elite) have the right to health, and "other" people (the marginalized and underserved populations) do not. It is here that the bioethical dimensions of the practice and industry are brought into a much sharper focus than could be achieved with more benign descriptors such as the term "medical travel."

MEDICAL TOURISM AND ECONOMIC DEVELOPMENT IN INDIA

The bioethical dimensions to medical tourism are particularly evident in the context of developing nations as destinations. India, with its heaving population, widespread poverty, and cavernous divides along the lines of caste, class, and religion, face critical health issues where social, cultural, and economic inequities are widening in terms of access, cost, and quality of healthcare. In rural areas, there are vast shortages of health practitioners and hospital beds to service the population. In urban areas, where there is a higher concentration of practitioners and services, the escalating costs in accessing these are driving many into crippling financial depression. In a country where almost a quarter of the local population go untreated for illness due to the indebtedness it causes, the aggressive promotion and expansion of commercial for-profit health for the comparatively wealthy, by governments and corporations, is a glaring mismatch of priorities that is difficult to ethically rationalize. However, forceful arguments of economic rationalism continue to drive both local and international support of the industry.

Dr Patel, a high-profile consultant surgeon in Mumbai, discussed the possible development opportunities for the Indian economy if medical tourism were to escalate in the predicted manner:

[It will] put us on the world map, I think. The world has considered us as a Third
World country; we still are. Let's face facts. This can change things. Definitely.
But the message is, we will now go to work, in all departments, in all faculties
of medicine. Very good, very well-trained doctors. Very well educated, not
generally the backward class I'm talking. By on large, the bulk of us are a very
good lot, well-trained lot.

Dr Patel was not alone in his optimism. Although media attention swings
between frenzied excitement and alarm about the prospects of medical tourism, the primary focus rarely shifts beyond the potential economic benefits
that will be derived from the industry. However, Dr Patel's reference to the
exclusion of the "backward class" also speaks volumes as to who will be
included as the ultimate benefactors of this emerging industry, and excluded,
both in the healthcare industry and the wider population.

The optimism and comparatively large share of media attention focused
on medical tourism over the last two decades belie the problematic data enu-
merating the industry, which is questionable at its very best. The monitors of
the market size have originated from private sources and estimates are more
likely indicative of the hopes of vested actors marketing the industry. Reports
on the global economic status of this service-based industry show wide dis-
crepancies, but industry reports have projected that the international industry
is worth as much as USD 85 billion and growing at a rate of 20% per annum.
Others have estimated that during 2015 more than 10 million patients sought
healthcare services in Asia, making up 80% of the global market (Lee and
Fernando 2015).

The private sector reported that only 10,000 foreigners annually obtained
medical services in India in the late 1990s. However, by 2001, the World
Health Organization (WHO) estimated that 50,000 people traveled to India
that year from Bangladesh alone to treat diseases that required specialist
care (Chanda 2001). Indian Government estimates have since indicated that
approximately 150,000 people travel to India for medical treatment annually;
however, it is likely that these numbers have significantly contracted during
the global coronavirus pandemic. In an interview in *The Indian Express*,
the president of the Apollo Group Hospitals acknowledged that somewhere
between 15 to 18% of the patients admitted to their Delhi hospital in 2005
were foreigners (Nazir 2006).

A survey conducted by the Indian Institute of Tourism and Travel
Management (IITTM) (2011) found that of 503 medical tourists in 35 hospitals across 17 Indian cities, the vast majority originated from African nations
(51%). The region with the next highest number of patients was the Middle
East (35%), and another 10% were from surrounding South Asian nations
(see figure 1.1). Despite the popularized notion of the movement of patients

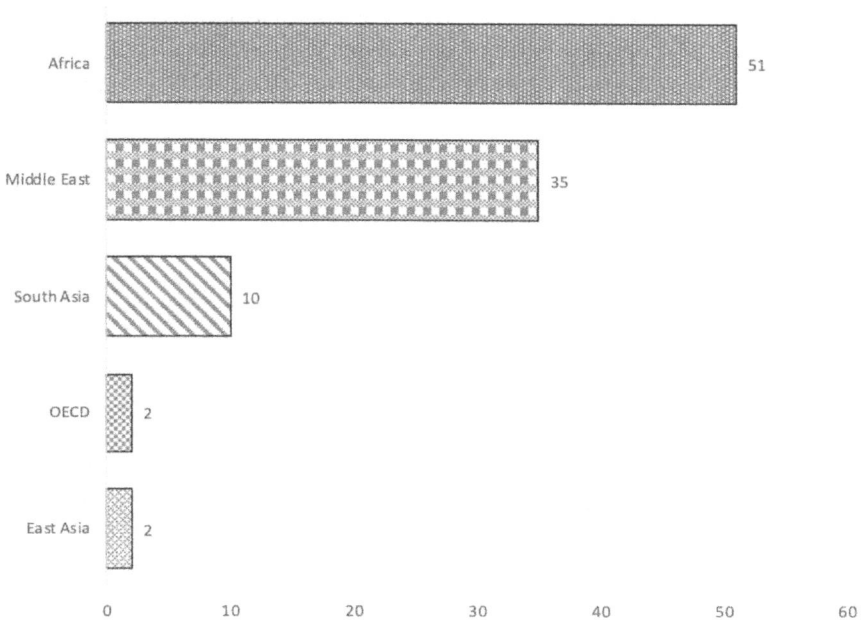

Figure 1.1   Medical Tourism Region of Patient Origin (%). *Source:* Image created by author. Data from Indian Institute of Tourism and Travel Management (2011).

from developed to developing nations, only 2% of respondents in the IITTM study were from OECD nations such as the United States, Canada, and the United Kingdom. This ethnographic study supports the IITTM survey, as the largest proportions of medical tourists in the five hospitals sites were from countries in surrounding regions, the majority originating from the Middle East and Africa. However, four out of the five hospitals in the research displayed trends of a gradual increase in patients from developed countries seeking healthcare services in Indian hospitals from 2007 onward (corresponding with the global financial crises).

The significance of the diaspora frequenting hospitals in India also emerged during fieldwork. Estimates provided by hospital administrators and consultants commenting on the high volume of diaspora accessing healthcare services indicate that this may be one of the larger segments undertaking this practice. Dr Desai, a consultant ophthalmologist across multiple clinics in the city explained that nonresident Indians (NRIs) made up a high proportion of his patients. He explained a typical scenario of NRI treatment,

Just a couple of weeks back I operated on a lady, a Person of Indian Origin, but settled in London. She was seen by at Moorfield's [Eye Hospital in London] and they told her that she had cataracts and that they needed to be operated [on]. She is related to a senior surgeon here [so] he called her down here, as a holiday, and in that interim period I operated on both her eyes over the span of 2 weeks. Then a week, or 10 days later she went back.

Dr Desai explained that although he sometimes treated POIs and NRIs from developed nations such as described above, a more regular patient base was sourced from NRIs based in the Middle East and in Africa, and that this segment of his "business" was increasing exponentially.

Dr Chopra, who was responsible for the administration of medical tourists in a large hospital in Mumbai explained that most medical tourists accessing their hospital were from Middle Eastern and African nations, with lower numbers from the United Kingdom and the United States. Dr Chopra noted that the main variation in patient origins since the hospital had opened was that they were progressively treating more patients from the United States.

Connell has also suggested more than 22% of Indian medical tourists are diasporic or NRI (Connell 2013). However, like most medical tourism in general, any attempt to enumerate rates of diaspora undertaking medical tourism is frustrated by the ad hoc processes used by different institutions to identify them. Of the five hospitals in this ethnography, all had different policies on their classification of medical tourists when collecting data. For example, only one of the five hospitals classified NRIs as medical tourists and two of the hospitals did not keep records of the residential status of patients at all. Further complicating matters, there is an additional category of residency status for people living outside of India with roots in the nation: person of Indian origin (PIO). PIOs are citizens of another nation but have held an Indian passport at some point or have parents or grandparents who were citizens of India, while NRIs are Indian citizens who do not reside in India. One of the hospitals collected data on both NRI and POI status, counting POIs as medical tourists, but not NRIs. Given these factors, it is unfeasible to gauge the actual number of NRI/POIs accessing the services of the hospitals; however, informants in all five hospitals reported that they regularly treated people in these categories.

GLOBAL STRUCTURAL HEALTHCARE
SERVICE INEQUITIES

The promotional advertising slogan "First World Treatment at Third World Prices" was broadly used in India in the early 2010s to attract medical tourists to the country. Although pithily contextualizing the distinct global inequities on which the industry is premised, it concisely articulates the vision sold, and understood, by Indian healthcare providers (i.e., medical value travel). These local conceptions of medical tourism in India in a global context reflect that of William Mazarella's (2003) ethnographic study of globalizing consumerism and the "commodity image" set in advertising agencies in Mumbai. Mazarella theorized that the national advertising produced in urban India reflects local "anxieties, commitments, and contradictions that animate that practice" (2003, 3).

The comparatively low cost of specialty medical procedures in India is arguably one of the biggest inducements for many prospective medical tourists. For example, if a resident of the United States required a heart bypass and was without sufficient health insurance, what would have cost them well over $100,000 in the United States could be accessed for around $10,000 in India in 2010. Given the high ratios of under-insured or uninsured in nations such as the United States, patients may have little choice than to travel outside of their home country to access nonelective treatments that are unaffordable at home.

Although often more low-key than the aggressive multi-million-dollar marketing campaigns from competitors in the private sector in Thailand, marketing tools employed by private healthcare groups and hospitals in India include hospital websites with specific "international patient" sections, affiliations with travel agencies and memorandums of understanding with internationally renowned research centers such as the Harvard Medical School. There are also many direct and indirect government policies and initiatives aimed at promoting the industry to international consumers.

The options available to individual "healthcare consumers" are rapidly multiplying and are capitalized on by private businesses, corporations, and governments looking to trade in on the lucrative healthcare market. For example, in 2008, the Delhi tourism board advertised "Medical Destinations" similar to that of other popular tourism destinations (Delhi Tourism and Transport Development Corporation 2008). Individuals could go online and select from a range of variables for their required surgery, choosing their preferences of price-point, geographical area, hospital, suite, and surgeon. This can then be packaged with a selection of postsurgical recuperative

Table 1.1   Cost of Medical Procedures in India vs the United States (USD)

Treatment	United States	India	Savings (%)
Heart bypass	$113,000	$10,000	91
Hip resurfacing	$47,000	$8,250	82
Liver Transplant	$500,000	$40,000	92
Orthopedic Surgery	$20,000	$6,000	70
Cosmetic Surgery	$20,000	$2,000	90

Source: data from Andrews (2012); Connell (2013); Ernst & Young (2006).

retreats at nearby five-star resorts located in beachside, mountain, or village areas.

When viewed through an equity and social justice lens, problems related to the assertive promotion healthcare services as global, consumable commodities come into far greater focus. Commodification of healthcare services have long been linked to cycles of inequality within populations due to several related processes. When healthcare processes are commodified, costs escalate, which ultimately places unsustainable financial burdens on the individuals and households that are the most disadvantaged. In turn, this leads to further exclusion from services and greater likelihood of impoverishment from the inability to work due to ill health. It also fosters the divisive delivery of healthcare services in terms of quality, reinforcing social segregation while increasing health disparities within populations. These factors, among others, have led to wide international acceptance that governments *should* fund at least an essential or basic level of healthcare, as the marketplace fails to accommodate for the negative impact on equity. As such, one of the foundational aims of this book is to locate medical tourism in a broader context that encompasses health equity and the commodification of healthcare systems, international development and health economics, local reconfigurations of the tertiary healthcare sector, and the mobility of the healthcare workforce.

Chapter 2

Medical Tourism and the Hypercommodification of Healthcare

During the past century, there have been historical shifts within the Indian healthcare system, transitioning away from a core reliance on traditional and indigenous systems of medicine toward that of state-sanctioned, market-led biomedicine. Contemporary understandings of what a health system is, or consists of, are not universal or widely agreed upon. The WHO (2015a) use an operational definition for health systems, where they posit it is composed of: (i) all the activities whose primary purpose is to promote, restore, and/or maintain health; (ii) the people, institutions, and resources, arranged together in accordance with established policies, to improve the health of the population they serve, while responding to people's legitimate expectations and protecting them against the cost of ill-health through a variety of activities whose primary intent is to improve health. Critical medical anthropology approaches view healthcare systems more holistically, incorporating all of the social relationships that are connected to both patient and healers (Baer, Singer, and Susser 2013).

The concept and study of global health has developed in alignment with understandings of globalization. It broadly focuses on health issues that reach beyond state boundaries, prioritizing issues of health equity across the globe. There are four interlinked areas commonly addressed by global health approaches of particular interest to the focus of this book. First is the examination of the effects of neoliberal economic and political shifts on healthcare systems in developing nations. The second is the influence and conduct of international organizations on healthcare systems in developing countries. Third, is the investigation of the relationship between the diminishing role of the public sector in healthcare systems and associated commodification of healthcare. The last, and most important to this context, is the impact of market-led healthcare models on healthcare for disadvantaged subpopulations.

Recent historical, social, and economic conditions have led to the Indian healthcare system's current configuration, with India emerging as one of the leading nations in the nascent medical tourism industry. Together, the international and local conditions have provided an opportunistic policy and commercial window for medical tourism to emerge. From a global perspective, international organizations led by the International Monetary Fund (IMF) and the World Bank pressured many developing nations toward the privatization and commercialization of their financial systems in the 1980s, which included sectors such as health and education. In India, a significant ideological shift emerged in the late 1980s, with neoliberal, market-led frameworks replacing earlier social-democratic conceptions of health and healthcare provision envisioned in the nation's early post-Independence era. This led to the incremental commodification of what has been (and largely continues to be) a fragmented, unregulated, and predominantly ad-hoc healthcare system, through a pro-privatization ethos that has permeated both political and social thought across the nation. This neoliberal turn has facilitated the emergence of a medical tourism industry in the nation, of which has both reinforced and hastened processes of healthcare commodification in the tertiary healthcare sector.

Understandings of commodification originate from Marxist thought, where it is viewed as the process by which the value of goods and services are transformed, with their social and political value being replaced by economic value. This framing aligns commodification with the capitalist processes of alienation, focusing on the transformation of goods into commodities through the products of human labor. Marx (1906) argued that "commodities possess an objective character as values only in so far as they are all expressions of an identical social substance, human labor, that their objective character as values is therefore purely social" (1906, 138–39). Appadurai, diverging from classical Marxist theories, has argued that any "thing" has the potential to be categorized as a commodity. Scheper-Hughes and Wacquant (2002, 94) extended this idea, noting that through an anthropological lens, the trade of commodities is more than "an emanation of individual needs, but a function of a variety of social practices and classifications."

The commodification of healthcare has invariably been referred to as the process by which healthcare services are recast as commodities, and patients as consumers, whereby the quality, cost, availability, and distribution of the "products" (the services) are dictated by the market (Pellegrino 1999; Henderson and Peterson 2002). Building on these theories, this book further situates medical tourism in the context of what I argue is a hypercommodified healthcare system in India. My conceptualization of hypercommodified healthcare builds on earlier definitions of commodified healthcare, expanding to capture all the material, social, and legal functions of healthcare services in the commodification process. In hypercommodified healthcare, the materiality of the buildings and land from where healthcare services are delivered, the human and mechanical labor used to deliver services, and the policies and laws that regulate healthcare and healthcare service delivery are all reconceived as processes that can be commodified. As these material, social, and legal functions are commodified, healthcare services are progressively valued for how they function in this hypercommodified healthcare system rather than any intrinsic value they may offer.

The medical tourism industry engages and interacts within the political, economic, and social processes that reproduce institutionalized complexes and structures of power that have led to broader systemic and systematic shifts. Healthcare hypercommodification has led to a broad spectrum of detrimental and debilitating effects for the most socioeconomically disadvantaged groups within the nation, signaling the harms that have already emerged from the persistence and expansion on this trajectory. By further unpacking some of these notions, this chapter contributes to the book's foundational argument that medical tourism, as an outcome of wider global and national healthcare commodification, has served to hasten and entrench both the processes of healthcare hypercommodification and consequent health disparities in India. An industry such as medical tourism must be considered within the broader formation of development in India; thus, this chapter presents the structural and systematic mise-en-scène of the book.

INDIA'S POPULATION DEMOGRAPHICS AND HEALTH STATUS

India is a nation of vast social, cultural, religious, political, and economic diversity, with 18 official languages spoken across 28 states and seven union territories. With a population of over 1.35 billion, India is home to almost 18% of the world's entire population. The population has multiplied five times since the start of the eighth century (see table 2.1) and is set to overtake China by 2025 (Singh 2014, 5). India is in the midst of rapid urbanization. Although the rural population more than doubled since the early 1960s, the urban population increased over three-fold over the same period (Yadav, Nikhil, and Pandav 2011, 3).

The combination of rapid urbanization and population growth in India has led to significant increases in population density, with national levels of 455 people per square kilometer (World Bank 2018). Notably, these densities are considerably higher in some regions, but particularly so in the larger metropolises of the country, such as Kolkata (24,306 per square kilometer), Mumbai (19,552 per square kilometer), and New Delhi (11,320 per square kilometer)

Table 2.1   Population Demographics in India

Indicator	Year	Data
Population (billion)	1985	0.784
	1995	0.963
	2005	1.148
	2015	1.31
	2019	1.366
Rural Population (% of total)	1985	58.78
	1995	55.16
	2005	50.85
	2015	46.09
	2019	44.29
Population Density (person per km2)	1985	263.8
	1995	324.2
	2005	386
	2015	440.7
	2018	454.9

Source: World Bank (2021a).

(Government of India 2011a). However, it is as yet unclear whether this rapid urbanization has reversed during the coronavirus pandemic.

In the nation's urban capitals, it is estimated that approximately one third of the population resides in slums (Yadav, Nikhil, and Pandav 2011). United Nations HABITAT (2015) characterizes slums as areas that are overcrowded, have insufficient access to safe water, poor sanitation, infrastructure, housing, and security of residential status.

India is in the midst of an epidemiological health transition with predictions that noncommunicable disease could overtake communicable diseases as the highest burden within the decade. The rising incidence of noncommunicable diseases has shifted the political and economic focus of the nation. India's health transition replicates global trends, where the majority of communicable diseases internationally have gradually become a problem experienced by only the poor and the vulnerable. Regardless, communicable diseases remain the highest cause of mortality and morbidity in many emerging and developing countries such as India, in spite of years of economic growth. India has one of the world's highest burdens of bacterial diseases, where in 2013 approximately 240,000 people died of tuberculosis and in even greater numbers from diarrheal diseases (World Health Organization 2014, 132).

The urban poor, in particular, carry a substantially higher burden of communicable diseases than other groups due to population health risk factors including poor access to sanitation, clean water, and medical treatment. Although official data reported by national agencies indicate that many of these factors have improved in recent decades, data is often inaccurate and unreliable. Many established slum areas are illegal or of unofficial status, so official government data describing these populations are often incomplete. Also, given the high levels of mobility of those living in slum areas, it is difficult to collect population level data that is inclusive of all residents.

Life expectancy, long seen as an indicative measure of a nation's health, remains low in India. Although, the life expectancy of the Indian population has increased dramatically from the time of India's Independence from 29 years (in 1947) to 69 years. Life expectancy in the nation is only now reaching that which many other developing countries achieved more than three decades ago yet remains considerably lower than the international average (73.4 years) (WHO 2020).

In 2016, the national child gender ratio was 87.7 females to 100 boys (see table 2.2), an imbalance that has worsened over the last five decades. Child sex ratios are often used as an indicator of gender imbalances in societies. In India, the preference toward boys is directly linked to the poor status of

Table 2.2   Development Indicators Over Time

Indicator	Year	Data
Life Expectancy at Birth (years)	1985	57
	1995	60
	2005	64
	2012	66
	2018	69
Child Sex Ratio	1961	976
(females per 1,000 males)	2001	927
	2011	919
	2013–15	900
	2016	877
Mean Years of Education	1985	1.9
	1995	3.3
	2005	4.0
	2010	5.4
	2018	6.4
Access to improved sanitation (%)	1990	18
	1995	21
	2005	30
	2012	36
	2015	40
Undernourished population (%)	1991	26
	1999	21
	2005	22
	2012	17
	2017	15

Source: Data from Government of India (2011a); United Nations Development Program (2014); World Bank (2014); Ritchie, H (2019); Government of India (2020).

women, embedded in economic, religious, and social relations. Further, state protections for women are often poorly enforced, including those related to property rights, inheritance laws, domestic violence, dowry prohibition, and crime against women. There are also reports of increasing unregulated sex selection practices across the nation facilitated by advances in high-tech biomedicine.

Education levels in India have rapidly improved over the course of the past three decades but remain low by international standards. On average, the majority of people still do not progress beyond (or complete) primary school (see table 2.2). Further, employment instability and vulnerability are another major factor impacting on the population. The vast and increasing majority of the working population is employed in the informal sector, estimated at upward of 80% of all employment outside of the agricultural sector. A gender bias operates within the informal sector, with women more likely than men to be working as informal workers. Jobs in the informal sector are generally lowly paid and insecure, offering little protection from labor laws, no health insurance or social protections and often operate within precarious labor arrangements. In the formal sector, employment in many industries is highly vulnerable to fluctuations in the international financial system. For example, it is estimated that approximately one million jobs were lost in the textile and apparel industries alone after the 2008 Global Financial Crisis (GFC) (United Nations Development Program 2014, 122).

However, India also has one of the fastest growing economies in the world, with a gross domestic product (GDP) growth rate that has hovered at around 7% for the last two decades. It is classed as one of the G-20 major economies and is a member of the BRICS nations, which are considered the top five emerging national economies of the world. Despite this, the population and human development indicators demonstrate overall trends of only negligible improvement over the last few decades. Even with these graduated improvements, the people of India are not faring well on an international scale. Based on the United Nations Development Project (UNDP) human development composite indicator, India ranks 135 out of 187 countries, placing it in the lower range of the United Nations classification of "medium human development."

Although there is considerable variation between and within states across India, table 2.3 provides an indication of India's overall health and development status in comparison to eight other nations. This set of countries all actively engage in and promote themselves as medical tourism destinations from vastly different regions, inclusive of the Americas, the Middle East, and Asia. Economically there is a high degree of diversity between (and within) these nations. Of these countries, India has the lowest gross national income (GNI) per capita and the worst population health outcomes.

Table 2.3 Comparison of Health and Development Indicators in Medical Tourism Destinations

Nation	GNI per capita (2011 PPP$)	Human Development Index	Life Expectancy at Birth 2018	Under 5 Years Mortality Rate (per 1,000 Live Births) 2018	Maternal Mortality Rate (per 100,000 Live Births) 2017	Tuberculosis Incidence (per 1,000 population)
Singapore	83,793	0.935	83.5	3	8	0
United Arab Emirates	66,912	0.866	77.8	8	3	1
United States	56,140	0.920	78.9	7	19	3
Malaysia	27,227	0.804	76.0	8	29	92
Mexico	17,628	0.767	75.0	13	33	23
Thailand	16,129	0.765	76.9	9	37	153
Costa Rica	14,790	0.794	80.1	9	27	10
Jordan	8,268	0.723	74.4	16	46	68
India	6,829	0.647	69.4	37	145	199

Source: United Nations Development Program (2019) World Health Organization (2020).

India's under five mortality rate is significantly higher than that of other nations engaging in medical tourism (see table 2.3). More children die in India than in any country in the world, accounting for one in every five child deaths across the globe (approximately 2.5 million deaths every year). Further, maternal mortality rates (MMR), often viewed as an indicator of a nation's gender imbalances, are extremely high in India. India had the worst MMR ranking of these medical tourism destinations, with 145 maternal deaths per 100,000 live births. India's 35,000 maternal deaths in 2017 accounted for over 10% of all maternal deaths globally ("WHO | Maternal Mortality: Levels and Trends" n.d.).

Low levels of health literacy, alongside lack of access to clean water and sanitation play a significant role in the ongoing proliferation of communicable disease, particularly in rural areas and for the urban poor. There were a number of formal and informal slums surrounding the apartment I lived in during fieldwork, in which I would wander through on most days in order to do my fruit and vegetable shopping and to catch the train, taxis, or autorickshaws. These slums were a mix of *kachcha* (temporary) and semi-*pukka* (more permanent) residences. The *kachcha* housing tended to be erected on and around building sites, where the workers would create their own spaces to live whilst working. The semi-*pukka* residences in one nearby slum were made from solid, longstanding materials in contrast to the mud, cardboard, and blue tarped constructions found in many other areas. The buildings were generally two-level, two-roomed residencies, attached to one another in long winding "lane-ways." Although some had electricity connections, they were unregulated, makeshift, and hazardous; commonly siphoned via illegal means from close by power mainlines. However, even in the semi-*pukka* slums there are far fewer infrastructural facilities available with low levels of sanitation and access to water. Particularly in the monsoonal season, the numbers of children and elderly people with diarrheal illnesses rise exponentially. The combination of the lack of health literacy and the poor infrastructure has damning effects on the health of slum populations, alongside the resultant financial burden caused by illness (i.e., inability to work, cost of treatment).

Structure of The Indian Healthcare System

Understandings of what a health system is, or consists of, are not universal or widely agreed upon. The WHO (2015) use an operational definition for health systems, composed of:

(i) all the activities whose primary purpose is to promote, restore, and/or maintain health.

(ii) the people, institutions, and resources, arranged together in accordance with established policies, to improve the health of the population they serve, while responding to people's legitimate expectations and protecting them against the cost of ill-health through a variety of activities whose primary intent is to improve health.

Biomedicine, widely known as allopathy in India, is the dominant medical system in the nation. However, it operates alongside multiple traditional and indigenous Indian systems of medicine. India has a long history of various systems of medicine and care practiced across the nation. The state-sanctioned traditional systems of medicine are Ayurveda, Yoga and Naturopathy, Unani, Siddha, and Homoeopathy, collectively referred to as AYUSH. The AYUSH medical systems hold significant and ongoing importance in the nation, particularly within the context of primary health. The independent Indian Ministry of AYUSH manages 3,277 AYUSH hospitals (with over 62,000 beds), over 24,000 dispensaries, with over 785,000 registered practitioners (Ministry of AYUSH 2021) across the nation.

The Ministry also manages six major research councils, two councils addressing regulation, education, and practice, three national pharmaceutical laboratories, 11 national institutes, and a drug manufacturing unit. Comparatively, it is estimated that there are 25,778 public and 43,486 private biomedical hospitals in India (Jaffrelot and Jumle 2020). Local health traditions (LHT), sometimes referred to as ethnomedicine or indigenous healing, are also widely practiced across the country and include an extensive range of heterogenous practices such as *marma chikitsa* and other forms of spiritual healing. Although generated over centuries, most LHT knowledge is dynamic, translated via oral means and practiced at a household level. However, there is a much higher reliance on the biomedical system, with only approximately 5% of the population relying solely on healthcare outside of biomedicine (National Statistical Office 2020, iii)

Like most healthcare systems internationally, India's existing healthcare system is arranged across three levels: primary, secondary, and tertiary. The highest proportion of curative care is delivered at the primary healthcare (PHC) level by the private sector. Although difficult to quantify, estimates indicate that approximately 80% of PHC services are delivered by the private sector where individuals generally pay directly for any PHC services they receive. Approximately a quarter of PHC practitioners are from the AYUSH medical systems, complemented by a significant proportion of other traditional healers (Rao, Nundy, and Dua 2005, 89). Although there has been increasing participation of private actors, including not-for-profits and philanthropists partnering with state governments in PHC provision, further corporate investment has emerged due to high demand, thus creating the potential for expansion in the area.

PHC services are publicly provided by Primary Health Centers, Subcenters and Dispensaries, and Community Health Centers. These facilities offer out-patient services, with limited in-patient services providing curative care, preventive care, and health promotion. Subcenters are often the first point of contact within the public healthcare system, with services in maternal and child health, family welfare, nutrition, immunization, and disease control (Mondal and Kanwal 2006). Most PHCs have only one medical officer on staff, with up to 14 other paramedical employees, and around 30 beds onsite. However, Community Health Centers usually have qualified medical professionals and specialists, acting as a referral center for more specialized care if required (Mondal and Kanwal 2006).

The political priority afforded to PHC in India has left secondary healthcare (SHC) largely neglected with deficiencies in funding, resources, and infrastructure. As a consequence, most SHC is provided by the private sector. The size of the sector is largely unknown due to poor data collection and inadequate sectoral regulation. The majority of services at this level are provided by what are known as "nursing homes," similar in function and size to district hospitals, accommodating 10 to 30 beds. Nursing homes are extremely underresourced and are widely cited as providing decidedly variable levels of care. Many healthcare workers in this sector have no formal medical qualifications (Das et al. 2012). Public sector SHC infrastructure includes the Employees State Insurance Scheme (ESIS) hospitals, district hospitals, maternity services, women and children's hospitals, psychiatric hospitals, contagious diseases hospitals, and medical education institutions (NHAC 2005).

The private sector also provides the majority of tertiary healthcare (THC) in India. The private THC sector has experienced rapid expansion in recent decades, where as many as 150 private corporate chains such as Apollo, Max, Fortis, and Escorts have established corporate hospitals mainly across the urban centers of the nation. Many of these are technologically driven, superspecialty, 100 plus bed facilities. There is also a large network of charitable (Trust) hospitals operating across the nation. In the absence of sufficient and reliable care in the public sector, charitable hospitals have provided a safety net for a vast number of the population, offering services at considerably lower costs than within corporate institutions. However, within the contemporary political and economic climate, Trust hospitals are struggling to maintain economic viability, leading to increases in the cost of services and shifts to their philanthropic ideology. These transformations are outlined in greater detail in chapter four.

Although governments (central, state, and municipal) own and operate leading hospitals such as the All India Institute Medical Sciences (AIIMS) institutions, Public-Private-Partnerships (P-P-P) are becoming the new norm, blurring the division between public and private healthcare delivery. State health corporations sponsored by the World Bank have founded collaborations between the public and private sector, where although the government may retain ownership of the hospital, the management of and equipment provision are contracted out to private companies. This has led to criticism from many Indian public health advocates, with doctors and hospital administrators voicing their concerns about the high levels of corruption that unremittingly plague the public THC sector.

Healthcare provided by the public sector is a joint responsibility, implemented over three levels of government: state, central, and municipal. However, approximately 75% of service delivery is executed at the state and municipal levels. The state governments are the primary providers of healthcare, also directing local government in health provision and programs. The central government is responsible for national standardization measures of health, allocating aid resources to states, funding various state-based programs, and providing health services for union territories that that are devoid of appropriate legislation. Both state and central governments jointly govern areas including family welfare and population control, quality control and standards for food, and pharmaceuticals and medical education.

The neglect of state Public Health Acts in India is demonstrative of the limited legislative controls within the public healthcare system. Public Health Acts are the formal legal structures regulating the delivery of public health services, but in most states in India, they have not been addressed or revised since pre-Independence. For example, Tamil Nadu's Public Health Act dates back to 1939 (National Sample Survey Organization 2006, 20).

Out-of-pocket Impoverishment

Internationally, spending on health is increasing at a faster rate than the rest of the global economy (GDP). In 2017 alone, international health expenditure was in excess of USD $7.5 trillion (Xu et al. 2018). On average, governments provide approximately half of the expenditure on health and out-of-pocket expenses cover around one-third of spending (WHO 2019). It is estimated that out-of-pocket spending forces over 100 million people into extreme poverty across the world on an annual basis.

In India, the government only contributes approximately a third of all healthcare spending. In Purchasing Power Parity (PPP), this accounts for a mere $68.73 per person, indicative of the abysmal state of the public healthcare system. Conversely, out-of-pocket spending coming directly from households is extraordinarily high, representing almost two-thirds of all healthcare expenditure (see figure 2.1).

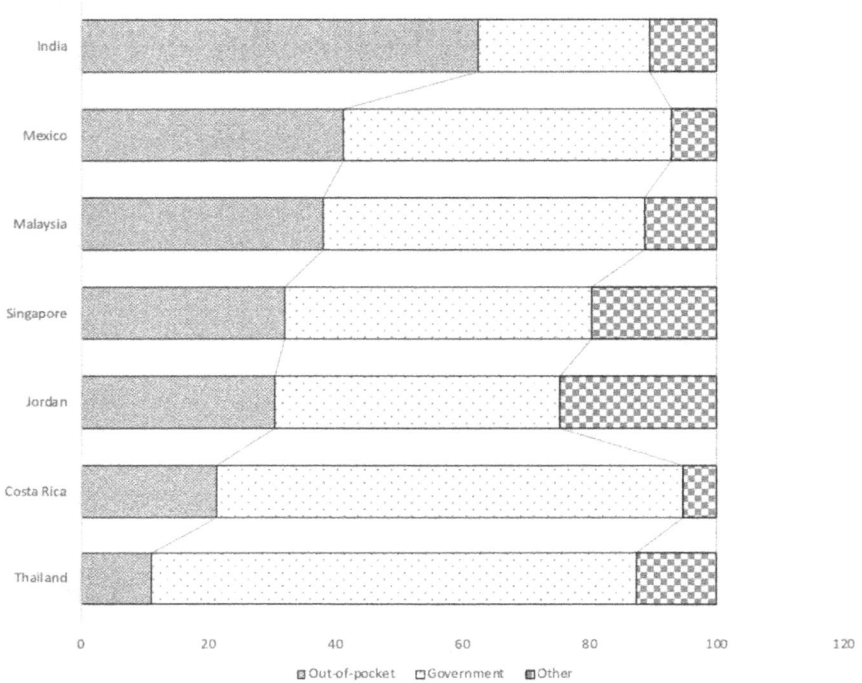

Figure 2.1   Source of Healthcare Expenditure (% of Total) 2017. *Source*: Image created by author. Data from the World Bank (2021).

Healthcare systems reliant on out-of-pocket spending create perverse financial incentives, causing severe financial hardship and impoverishment for individuals and households when someone falls ill. The large disparities between health indicators in developed and developing countries can be viewed through the lens of the inverse care law, which refers to how the accessibility of healthcare operates in a relationship inverse to need (UNDP 2005, 26). Further, the differences in healthcare expenditure follow a similar pattern, as countries with the highest need are generally the most under-funded.

The Rise of Biomedicine in India

Medical pluralism has flourished in India for centuries. As noted earlier, biomedicine is now the dominant medical system of the nation, however, it still operates in conjunction with multiple traditional and indigenous Indian systems of medicine. Although medicine in India had already started to move away from magico-religious to empirico-rational therapies between 400 BC

India   68.7

Jordan   339.0

Thailand   510.7

Mexico   533.5

Malaysia   576.2

Costa Rica   927.8

Singapore   2,058.3

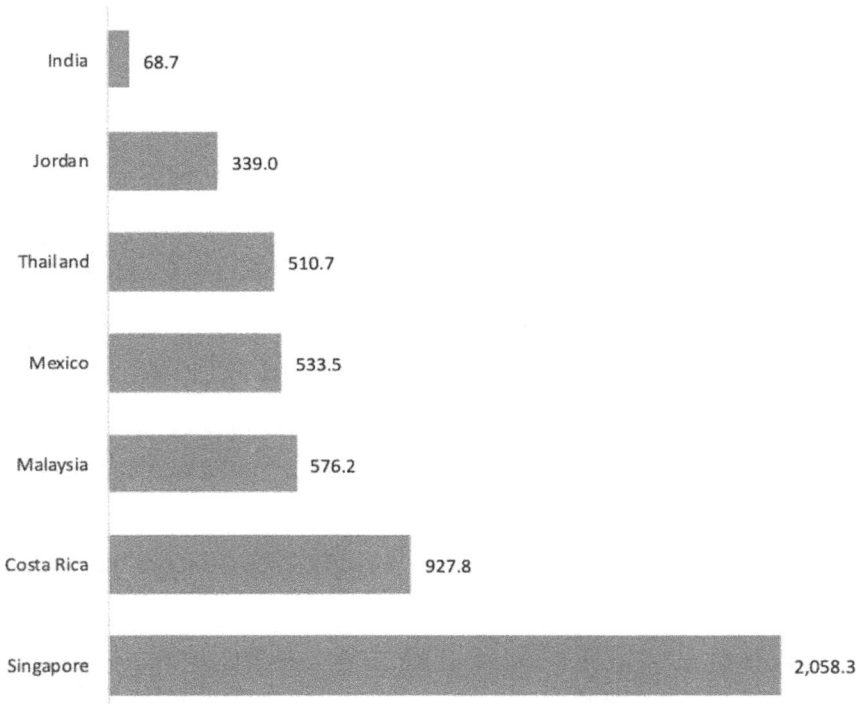

Figure 2.2   Government Per Capita Spending on Health (2017). *Source*: Image created by author. Data from World Bank (2021).

and 1500 AD, some regard the penetration of biomedicine into India as one of the most detrimental and pervasive legacies of the British colonial rule (Arnold 1993; Banerji 1981). The colonial introduction of new medical systems in the so-called global South has triggered complex and contextually specific outcomes in different nations. This is due to the highly interconnected relationships between the delivery of healthcare services to a population and the wider political economy, social functioning, and cultural systems of a nation. In India, many health cultures were well established and effective in the alleviation of illness and promotion of good health prior to colonization. However, during British rule, many of these health cultures deteriorated. It is important here to note that there are significant variations of how "good health" is understood from the perspectives of different medical systems.

In the latter years of colonization, the British established medical colleges to train Indian doctors in biomedicine, however, British doctors continued to dominate senior appointments in the Indian Medical Service up until India's Independence. By this time, Christian missionaries had become highly active advocates of biomedical health, with many groups running dispensaries and educational facilities to train local nurses in urban regions (see chapter 5 for further details).

Post-independence, India's first Prime Minister, Jawaharlal Nehru, was a staunch advocate of democracy and socialism (Desai 1987), introducing the notion of democratic economic planning in India. In March 1950, the Planning Commission prepared the first in a long line of Five-Year-Plans (FYP), outlining India's path to development, which continue to this day. From the outset, these plans aimed "to build up by democratic means a rapidly expanding and technologically progressive economy and a social order based on justice and offering equal opportunity to every citizen" (Government of India Planning Commission 2002, n.p.).

Nehru was staunchly opposed to private monopolies and maintained that basic and heavy industries should be kept within the public realm. "Nehruvian" politics prevailed within national economic planning for many years, with ongoing reliance and dependence on the central government for national macroeconomic structure, management, and delivery. The Central government controlled subsidies, tariffs, and quota allocations. Although the British initiated many of these features during colonial rule, the first Indian government extended and reinforced these controls. The first four decades after India's Independence was dominated by extensive planning regimes, with an emphasis on the public sector and investment in basic and heavy industries.

In these early years post India's Independence, the country's Bhore Report (Bhore 1946) was highly influential in the development, structure, and approach for the nation's healthcare system. The report espoused a social medicine approach to healthcare for the nation, recommending a publicly managed and resourced system that would integrate both curative and preventative approaches. However, the Bhore Report did not include the indigenous medical systems in this "comprehensive" approach, stating:

> It was not until the middle of the 19th century that medical science became firmly on a secure foundation . . . we can say with truth that 95% of the total corpus of knowledge with regard to the working of the human body has been obtained within the lifetime of men who are still with us...science is one and indivisible (Bhore 1946, 455–56).

This divisive framing of biomedicine as scientific medicine relegated traditional and indigenous systems of medicine as "cheap," backward, and inferior. Metaphors of progress were associated with biomedicine, contextualizing the system within the paradigm of modernity. In particular, Western conceptualizations of "modernity" arose from the seventeenth century, firmly positing assumptions that the processes of "industrialization, urbanization, commodification, rationalization, differentiation, bureaucratization, the expansion of the division of labor, the growth of individualism and state formation processes" (Featherstone 1995, 12) are all features of one global, unitary history. However, it is important to understand that modernity's emancipatory features such as human rights, democracy, and prosperity are often the primary features championed, drawing attention away from its imperialistic underpinnings. The notion of progress forms a central and recurrent aspect of modernity, with science and technology heralded as the solution to most social problems (Escobar 2004). Through the lens of ecofeminism, Mies and Shiva (1993) maintain that science as a knowledge system is intrinsically patriarchal and colonial and is organized in opposition to nature. They contend this manifests across multiple levels, but is most evident in practices such as biotechnology and reproductive technology.

From the 1960s through to the mid-1980s, signs of liberalization emerged in the Indian economy, including the reduction of regulatory barriers in particular areas such as foreign investment in multiple sectors. The 1980s saw a major shift in policy direction toward the neoliberal "efficiency" approach; the beginnings of which can be seen in the National Health Policy 1982 (Directorate-General of Health Services India Ministry of Health and Family Welfare 1983), formally acknowledging the role played by the private health sector for the first time.

The neoliberal efficiency approach gained international traction with the advent of the Structural Adjustment Programs (SAP) introduced in many developing countries in the late 1980s and early 1990s by the World Bank and the IMF. In a rejection of earlier Keynesian approaches that encouraged state intervention in the economy, the SAPs were underpinned by neoliberal principles of deregulation and free trade. The key aim of the SAPs was to reduce public investment and management of a range of services in areas such as health and education. In policy terms, this neoliberal approach was implemented via significant reductions in public spending and pro-privatization regimes, which were argued to make the sectors more economically efficient.

Before the 1980s, the World Bank rarely offered loans specifically targeted to health. However, its first report on Financing Health Services in Developing Countries outlined its initial policy and strategy regarding market reforms in health systems (World Bank 1987). The subsequent release of the World Development Report: Investing in Health expanded on these strategies, arguing that the most significant problem of healthcare systems in developing nations was the misuse and misallocation of government health resources (World Bank 1993). While noting that the improved health of populations is integral to economic development, as this "permits the use of natural resources that had been totally or nearly accessible because of disease" (World Bank 1993, 3–4), the report warned that public health resources should be confined to an essential clinical package of curative care for the poor. Any curative services beyond a basic level were categorized as goods to be provided and regulated by the market. The significance of this report was dual-fold, in that it indicated a shift in international health leadership from the World Health Organization (WHO) to the World Bank and widely informed the direction and scope of health reform in developing countries. The report also set the agenda for governments implementing the health reforms, particularly those reliant upon World Bank funding.

The effects of SAPs were widely critiqued from the late 1980s onward, particularly from the perspective of the negative impact of SAPs on the most disadvantaged populations within nations. Stiglitz, an outspoken critic of the IMF and former chief economist of the World Bank, has argued that although the IMF was initially established on the basis of providing stability to counteract global market imperfections and failures, "it now champions market supremacy with ideological fervour" (Stiglitz 2002, 17). In reference to the SAPs, Stiglitz contends that at worst they have "led to hunger and riots in many countries" (2002, 24) and at best have led to slow, temporal economic growth that has unduly benefitted the wealthy, often at the expense of the poor. Other scholars have also imparted exacting critiques of the measures introduced by the IMF via their conditional loans offered to developing nations (Stuckler and Basu 2009). Case studies, particularly across South Asia, have illustrated how SAPs undermine the comprehensive nature of primary healthcare, encouraging ineffective vertical health programs (Bennett 2001; Khan 2001; Qadeer 2002). Regardless, neoliberal efficiency principles have guided systematic healthcare reform across the globe, with the primacy of the IMF and the World Bank's influence on health policy only increasing over time.

When Rajiv Gandhi came to power in India in 1984, he implemented a set of macroeconomic adjustment policies, and consequent growth levels of over 8% were recorded in 1985. However, over the course of the next decade, external foreign debt had doubled (Denoon 1998). By 1987, it was recognized in the National Statistical Survey Organization 42nd Round that over 70% of the nation's populace were using some form of private healthcare (Lefebvre 2009).

In early 1991, India's foreign exchange reserves were at an all-time low, falling below USD $1 billion. The inflation rate also rose exponentially, reaching 16.7% at its peak (Agarwal 2006). With the promise of substantial debt relief from the World Bank and the IMF in the form of additional loans, in May of 1991, an SAP was introduced in India. In December 1991, a $500 million Structural Adjustment Loan (SAL) was approved by the World Bank, which was closed in 1993 (Agarwal 2006, 649). The IMF also approved two stand-by arrangement loans (SBAs) across the same period, the first in January 1991 for $551 million and the second in October 1993 for $1,656 million (World Bank 1996). India has, in fact, received the highest proportion of SAP loans in the world (World Bank 2021).

One of the first after-effects of the SAPs was the Indian Government's implementation of the New Economic Policy (NEP) in late 1991, which extended upon earlier macroeconomic adjustments. These policies sought to implement fundamental changes in the operation of the nation's economy, including devaluing the rupee; reduction of government controls over national industry; sale of public enterprises through different measures of privatization; dramatic cutbacks in government expenditure in the social sectors; and additional encouragement of foreign direct investment (FDI). The most significant outcome for the health sector was immediate, with extreme reductions to the central health budget, mainly via reduction of grants to state public health and disease control programs. Between 1974 and 1982 central grants to the states made up 19.9% of state health expenditure but, as a direct result of the SAP, grants fell to 3.3% in 1992 to 1993 (Purohit 2001). These reductions in spending were implemented across all centrally funded health programs (see table 2.4). Although the reduction of grants had an impact on all states across the nation, it had more marked consequences upon less resourced states, as they were unable to compensate for the shortfall through the use of local resources.

Alongside the central budget cuts and national economic downturn of the early 1990s, an ever-growing demand for medical services led to the proliferation of health services within the private sector, although it was still mainly limited to cities in the south of the country (Baru 2001). At the same time, regulations were lowered for foreign direct investment (FDI), which opened the floodgates for partnerships between foreign investors with Indian healthcare providers, particularly in corporate hospital groups (Denoon 1998). Between 1991 and 1997, the Foreign Investment Promotion Board approved US$100 million of FDI in the healthcare sector (Purohit 2001).

Table 2.4   Health Expenditure Met by Central Grants

Division of Health	1984–85	1992–93
Medical & Public Health	6.73	3.7
Public Health	27.92	17.17
Prevention & Disease Control	41.47	18.5
Family Welfare	99	88.59

Source: Data from Purohit (2001, p. 87).

THE ENDURING GLOBAL AGENDA OF
HEALTH COMMODIFICATION

The World Trade Organization (WTO) is another global agenda setting international institution that has had a high degree of influence over the structural framing of international and national health policies. The WTO governs global trade, brokering agreements dealing with goods, services and intellectual property, aiming to reduce nation state-based barriers to trade. In January 1995, the 160 member countries of the WTO committed to a time frame regarding their first trade agreement pertaining to services: the General Agreement on Trade in Services (GATS). In a briefing note, The WTO Secretariat rationalized the inclusion of health services in the GATS by asserting the efficiency that liberalization could bring the sector:

> While health and social services have long been considered as (a) non-tradeables to be provided by (b) public institutions, there has been a change in policy perception in a number of countries. More efficient transport and communication technologies have enhanced the mobility of both professionals and consumers and enabled the use of new modes of supply (telemedicine), overturning traditional concepts of space and distance. At the same time, new forms of private sector involvement have opened breaches for increased domestic and foreign participation. (World Trade Organization 1998, 2)

This commitment held that negotiations for GATS would commence in 2000 and that WTO members would have ongoing negotiations in order to progressively expand upon their commitments. The GATS is made up of three sections: (1) general obligations applicable to all GATS signatories; (2) rules pertaining to particular sectors; and (3) specific obligations for individual nations with regard to market access.

In developing countries, services have become one of the largest contributors to the GDP, where between January and March 2006, India's service sector made up 54.7% of the GDP (Hong 2000). This has grown considerably since the implementation of the SAPs in the early 1990's, where from 1985 to 1990, the service sector consisted of only 40.6% of the GDP (Ministry of Finance 2006). Within India's GATS schedule, the government has agreed to particular obligations with regard to hospital services, providing that hospitals are able to be developed with foreign equity contributions of up to 51% (Kumar 2006). To date, only 27% of the 160 member countries have also done so.

The GATS are founded upon two general provisions, being the "Most Favored Nation" and the "National Treatment." These two provisions denote the way a country is obligated to operate with regard to their treatment of other countries. The Most Favored Nation provision refers to the principal that any favorable treatment given to a foreign country requires the same treatment to be made available to all other GATS signatories. The National Treatment provides all companies operating offshore, but originating from a GATS signatory nation, must be given the same treatment as a national company. These provisions can be enforced by the WTO through their dispute resolution panel, where they are able to impose trade sanctions against any member countries found to be operating in noncompliance. Under the GATS, health is one of the 12 listed services. There are four different modes of health services covered: cross-border trade; consumption abroad; commercial presence; and movement of persons. Medical tourism falls within the second mode of the GATS. The GATS have drawn critique for a range of reasons, including the way the agreements restrict "the range of options that state and federal regulators and legislative bodies can employ to regulate the health sector and implement healthcare reforms" (I. Gupta 2004), which also serves to promote private over public interests.

The GATS negotiations were undertaken behind closed doors, without public scrutiny or debate and with no public disclosure required prior to their finalization. The methods and means of negotiation avoided interrogation, with questions of power and influence wielded by different nations remaining unclear. In a de-restricted joint communication to the WTO, delegates from India, Cuba, the Dominican Republic, Haiti, Kenya, Pakistan, Peru, Uganda, Venezuela, and Zimbabwe raised concerns regarding the commitments of developing nations comparatively to OECD nations under the GATS (World Trade Organization 2001). These nations collectively argued that opening services in the social sector to market forces through "re-regulation" was "fundamentally incompatible" to their responsibility to provide basic services to vulnerable sectors of their populations, who would otherwise have no access due to inability to pay market prices. The delegates also questioned the rationale of marketizing and commoditizing "common/public" resources in developing countries, when experience has shown that this generally leads to further barriers to access for much of the population. They further noted.

The experience of several developing countries with structural adjustment already shows that large segments of the population are having serious difficulties gaining access to basic commodities and services at prices they can afford" (WTO 2001, 5). The communiqué also addressed the proposal for continued regulation in areas where "technical standards and licensing in certain professional services, is used to effectively restrict entry by developing countries in the industry. (WTO 2001, 5)

Ongoing neoliberal reforms that hasten the commodification of India's healthcare system have continued in recent decades. For example, in December 2014, the Indian Government announced it would cut its five billion dollar public health funding by approximately 20% (Mudur 2015). Even prior to this announcement, the government had contributed only 1.3% of its annual GDP to health, lagging significantly behind other emerging economies across the globe. The previous (Congress) government had promised to increase health spending to 3% of the GDP, but in the face of a large tax revenue deficit, the Bharatiya Janata Party (BJP) government unveiled its New Health Policy (NHP) with the concurrent substantial reduction in expenditure. The BJP pitched this as an outcome of devolving greater national tax revenues to the states, implying the consequent effect of increased state spending and responsibility for the sector.

In 2019, the Indian government launched the national Ayushman Bharat scheme, the world's largest public health insurance scheme, aimed at delivering universal healthcare by targeting the lowest socioeconomic households across the nation (around 40% of the population). The scheme provides insurance coverage for families to access secondary and tertiary healthcare services through a network of both public and private providers. However, given the scheme's aim to provide universal healthcare, the resource focus on secondary and tertiary healthcare, as opposed to primary healthcare, is problematic. Achieving universal healthcare is one of the World Health Organization's key targets for the sustainable development goals and is generally achieved by investing in and strengthening primary healthcare. Instead, the Ayushman Bharat scheme diverts resources for health infrastructure away from the primary sector toward the tertiary sector. Given the already disproportionate expansion of the private tertiary sector of the past few decades, this mass injection of insurance capital only serves to further distort and weaken the healthcare system.

Equity Impacts of the Commodification of Healthcare

To empirically illustrate the widely detrimental impact of the collective macroeconomic reforms to the Indian healthcare system on different socioeconomic classes, I conducted analyses on historical datasets drawn from a series of Indian national household surveys to highlight the widening equity gaps for different socioeconomic sectors of the population before and after the introduction of the SAPs and NEP in the early 1990s. I have included analyses of multiple general economic indicators to trace patterns of inequity emerging over time using Monthly Per Capita Expenditure (MPCE) as a measure of socioeconomic status.

Although there is limited reliable data related to shifts in the general pricing of healthcare services over time in India, analyzing data on the illnesses

Table 2.5   Categorization of Socioeconomic Groups

Socioeconomic Group	MPCE (USD) Urban	MPCE (USD) Rural	Urban Population (%)	Rural Population (%)
Lowest	< 300	< 425	11.3	11.4
Lower middle	300–420	425–664	24.5	27.5
Upper middle	421–615	665–1120	34.3	33.0
Highest	> 615	> 1120	29.9	28.1

Source: Data from National Sample Survey Organization (2006, p. 20).

going untreated due to financial difficulty before and after the SAP provides a good indication of the impact of the ongoing neoliberal reforms on the population's access to healthcare services. The increased cost of accessing healthcare after the SAPs were introduced led to greater inaccessibility for both urban (11%) and rural (9%) populations (see figure 2.3). In 2004, this pattern continued in rural areas, with a further 4% of the population unable

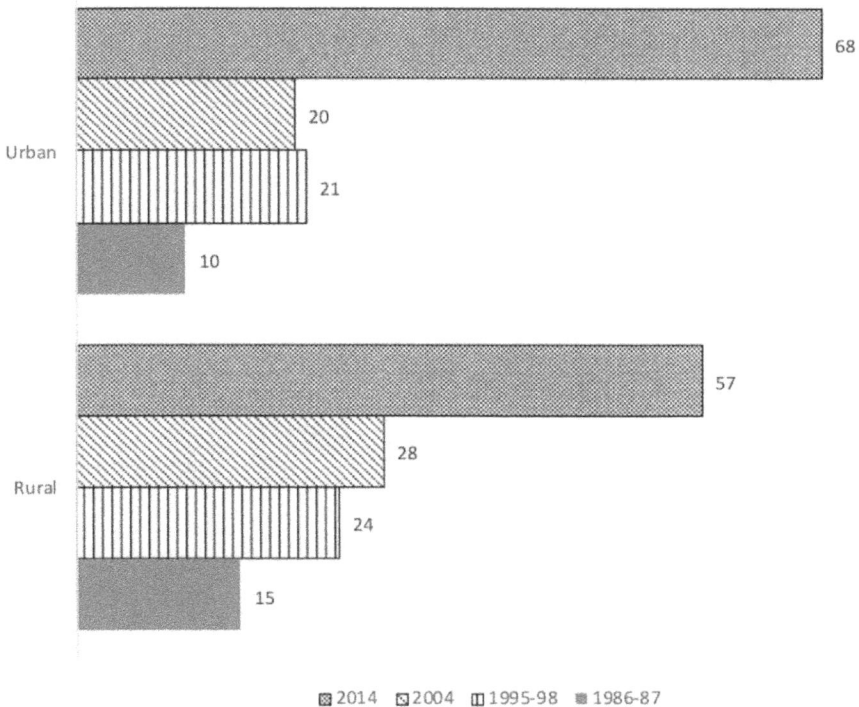

Figure 2.3   Untreated illnesses due to Financial Difficulties (%). *Source*: Image created by author. Data accessed from the National Sample Survey Office (2006, 2014).

to access medical care between 1995–96 and 2004. These trends increased exponentially during the following decade (2004–2014), with over half of the rural population and more than two-thirds of the urban population going untreated when ill due to the cost (see figure 2.4).

Further, those in lower socioeconomic groups were significantly less likely to go untreated when ill. figure 2.4 further demonstrates how the lowest socio-economic groups in both urban and rural regions are approximately twice as unlikely go untreated than those in the highest socioeconomic bracket. Also, people living in rural areas are less likely to access treatment for illness than those in urban areas.

In both rural and urban areas, those in the lowest socioeconomic groups were spending less per month on all aspects of life than the price to treat an average illness over the course of 15 days. However, for the wealthiest 25% of the population (the highest MPCE group), medical costs were only a little

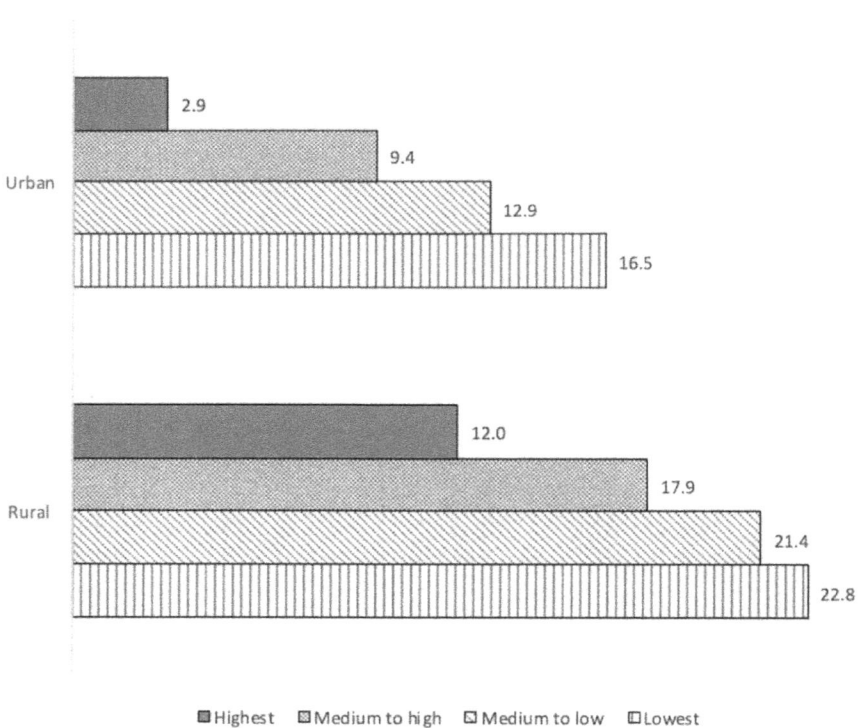

Urban
- 2.9
- 9.4
- 12.9
- 16.5

Rural
- 12.0
- 17.9
- 21.4
- 22.8

■ Highest   ▨ Medium to high   ▧ Medium to low   ▢ Lowest

Figure 2.4   Untreated Illnesses by Socioeconomic Status 2004 (%). *Source*: Image created by author. Data accessed from NSSO National Sample Survey Organisation (2006, p. 30).

more than third of their average monthly spending for those in rural areas and a quarter of the per capita expenditure for those in urban areas.

As shown in figure 2.5, the comparative financial burden of outpatient illness also depreciates as socioeconomic status rises. This is a stark example of the impact of socioeconomic inequity of healthcare access in India.

The escalation of out-of-pocket costs related to accessing healthcare services has led to significant indebtedness for people living in both rural and urban areas, with those in the lower expenditure groups becoming more highly indebted by medical treatment. This decreases sharply for the two higher groups accordingly.

Escalating costs related to accessing medical care are the second highest cause of indebtedness in rural India. It is estimated that in 2011–12 alone, 50 to 60 million people were pushed into poverty by out-of-pocket medical

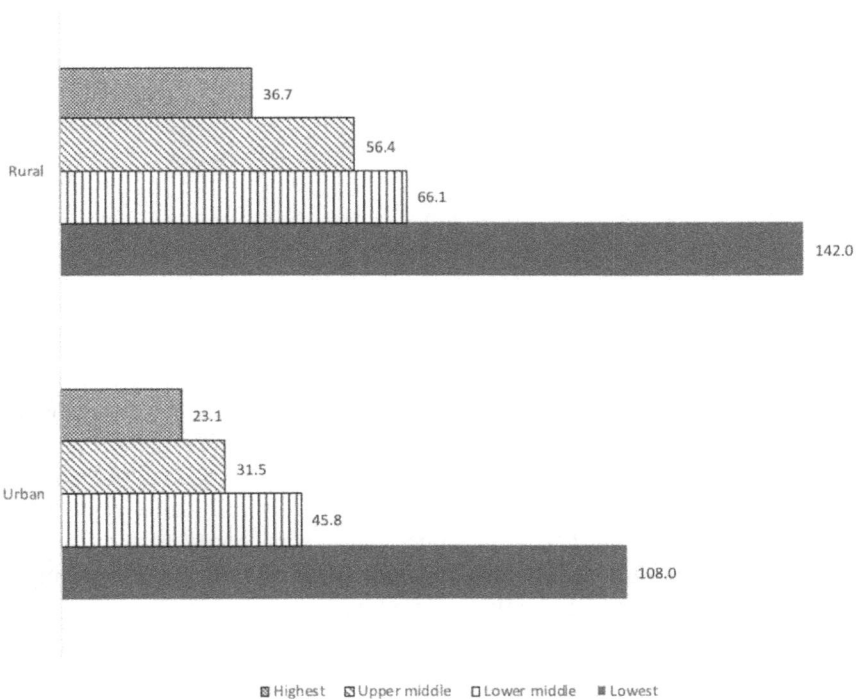

Figure 2.5   **Average Cost of Outpatient Hospitalization as a Percentage of Income (2004) by Socioeconomic Status.** *Expenditure includes both private and public costs for medical services alongside other related expenditure. *Total cost of non-hospitalized treatment over the course of 15 days, inclusive of all medical and other expenditure incurred as a result of the illness such as transport, accommodation, etc., but does not include household loss of earnings. *Source*: Image created by author. Data sourced from National Sample Survey Office (2006).

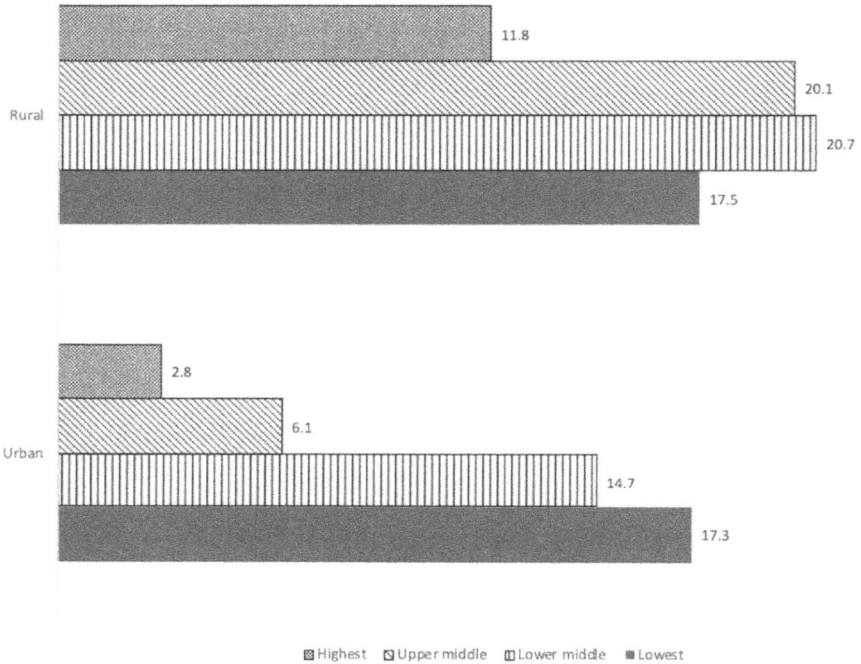

Figure 2.6 has the following values:

Rural: 11.8, 20.1, 20.7, 17.5

Urban: 2.8, 6.1, 14.7, 17.3

☒ Highest   ☒ Upper middle   ☒ Lower middle   ■ Lowest

Figure 2.6   Medical Treatment Causing Indebtedness by MPCE (%) 2004. *Source*: National Sample Survey Office (2006).

expenses (Selvaraj et al. 2018). The rural disadvantage is further compounded by the shortage of healthcare workers and hospitals located in rural regions. Although over 65% of India's population live in rural regions, more than 80% of biomedical doctors and more than 60% of hospitals are located in the urban centers (Selvaraj et al. 2018). In some states, particularly in the northern regions of the nation, the rural disadvantage is far more acute. For example, in the state of Bihar, there is only one medical doctor per 40,000 people.

These data highlight the further potential damaging effects of channeling resources into the medical tourism industry, due to its urban concentration and higher cost of services, being affordable only for middle to higher class Indian nationals.

Combined, these data present a grave account of India's position comparatively to other nations engaging in medical tourism, pointing to some of the critical health and health system issues faced by the nation. Many of the insufficiencies of the public health system in India can be traced directly to the paucity of public funding and reliance on households to pay for the cost of their own healthcare. With such a heavy reliance on individual out-of-pocket spending, the increasing costs of accessing healthcare have had an immeasurable impact on the predominantly income poor, and highly vulnerable populace. Even with the implementation of the Ayushman Bharat insurance program, critics have noted that the cap on payments for services does not sufficiently protect the poor from paying exorbitant additional fees that are not covered by the scheme. In this context, promoting a new industry such as medical tourism should be approached with a high level of caution, particularly in the absence of complementary regulatory or policy mechanisms safeguarding the population's access to affordable and safe healthcare.

COMMODIFIED HEALTHCARE AND
ECONOMIC EXCLUSION

Media, government, and private sector discourse often maintains that medical tourism will improve the public healthcare system and health status of the population in destination countries. Explanations of how this will be achieved rarely go beyond rhetoric, employing the widely critiqued "trickle-down" concept. Trickle-down theory, in the context of medical tourism, is generally applied via assertions that the economic growth derived from medical tourists will be siphoned back into hospitals and infrastructure, improving the technology, equipment, and increasing employment opportunities, benefiting the population at large. However, what is not acknowledged in these arguments is that the hospitals treating medical tourists are already high-end, elite institutions, and the hospitals requiring the most capital input, such as older Trust hospitals, public hospitals, and nursing hospitals, do not receive any financial benefit from medical tourism. Similarly, tourism more broadly, has long been posited as a driver of economic development for developing destination countries (de Kadt 1979), alongside corresponding cynicism related to the negative impacts tourism can have on local populations of host nations (Murphy 1985; Di Giovone 2009).

Another similar argument raised is that if "high-end" medical tourism hospitals expand, they may provide greater employment opportunities. Yet again, this may be the case for well-educated, trained, and elite healthcare professionals, but these benefits are less likely to flow through to the general Indian population. Further, it is yet again the elite hospitals and wealthy patients that benefit from any increases to the healthcare workforce, rather than the public sector where the need is the greatest.

The high-end biotechnology and specialized nature of medical tourism in India brings with it associations with modernism, placing it in prominently and positively in the public eye, serving as an example of a nation's general

Table 2.6   Untreated Medical Illness (%)

| | 1986–1987 | | 1995–1996 | | 2004 | |
Cause	Rural	Urban	Rural	Urban	Rural	Urban
Illness not seen as serious	75	81	52	60	32	50
Financial difficulties	15	10	24	21	28	20
Other	5	6	10	12	24	25
No medical facility	3	0	9	1	12	1
Lack of faith	2	2	4	5	3	2
Long waiting time	0	1	1	1	1	2

Source: Data from National Sample Survey Organization (2006, p. 20).

Table 2.7   Socioeconomic Variations in the Cost of Hospitalization (Rs)

| Expenditure | Rural | | | Urban | | |
Group	Public	Private	Difference (%)	Public	Private	Difference (%)
Low	2,597	5,287	50.88	1,993	5,928	66.38
Lower middle	2,543	5,972	57.42	2,680	6,619	59.51
Upper middle	3,137	6,540	52.03	4,180	9,682	56.83
Highest	4,872	9,306	47.65	9,588	17,703	45.84

Source: Data calculated from National Sample Survey Organization (2006, 27).

development. However, this refocusing only serves to further distort national health priories, drawing attention away from faltering public health systems and public health.

Another "trickle-down" argument posed is that the economic growth generated by medical tourism would result in an overall increase of national income, creating greater equity in access by allowing more of the population access to private care. However, this macro analysis fails to acknowledge those included and excluded from these benefits at large. Further, government promotion, concessions, and incentives directed toward the medical tourism industry must be challenged in contexts where public health expenditure is consistently reduced.

Medical tourism serves to reinforce a dual-tiered, market-led health system, consisting of a high-quality and high-priced sector catering to international patients and middle- to upper-class nationals; and a resource constrained, lower quality sector that is unable to serve the majority of the local population (Chacko 2005; Lautier 2008). Although medical tourism may benefit the elite of the nation and world, it is highly detrimental to the majority of the population. Invoking the inverse law of care, medical tourism directs healthcare resources away from those in the most need. The industry provides no panacea for economic development in India, and its ongoing promotion and delivery can only serve to widen the already vast social and health inequities evident across the nation.

CONCLUSION

India's early Bhore Report created a blueprint for the comprehensive delivery of healthcare across the nation, holding notions of equity as a high priority. However, from this time there has been a significant shift in priorities in the sector, where through a process of hypercommodification, the Indian health-care system has become one of the most privatized, inequitable systems in the world.

As healthcare services in India are ever more commodified, the notion of equity becomes further removed. Evidence from government, international organizations, and other sources all highlight the disproportionate funding that is directed to the private sector, primarily through individual out-of-pocket spending. This market-driven healthcare model operates in the context of a population with high levels of income poverty, sparse health insurance, and extensive out-of-pocket expenditure. Medical expenditure is the second highest cause of indebtedness in rural areas. Although 65% of India's population lives in rural areas, more than three quarters of the nation's biomedical doctors and hospital beds are located in urban centers. Further, approximately 75% of specialists work solely in a private sector that is already concentrated in the cities.

As illustrated in this chapter, the cost of medical treatment in India has consistently escalated over and above the level of inflation from the early 1990s, aligning with the introduction of neoliberal reforms under the SAP and subsequent NEP. Mounting medical costs impact most severely on the poorest 25% of the population, where the average cost of treating a non-hospitalized illness is more than the combined total of all other household expenses (MFHW 2006, 2004, 2006). In this economic climate, the costs of further commodifying one of the most highly privatized healthcare systems in the world are manifold. The heavy reliance on the private sector to deliver healthcare underscores the tensions between health as a human right and its neoliberal, capitalist framing as a commodity. In a nation the size of India, the social implications are vast and tyrannical in their impoverishing underpinnings. The conflicts emerging within the healthcare workforce are merely one indication of the evident contradictions. It is an emerging disaster, with the battle lines drawn, belittling global efforts to place health rights at the fore-front of an international agenda. Impacts from the shortcomings of India's healthcare system outlined in this chapter have already been highlighted during the global Covid-19 pandemic, driving vast swathes of the population into further impoverishment due to the costs associated with accessing private healthcare (Jaffrelot and Jumle 2021).

The emergence of medical tourism has also created an imbalance between regulation and the promotion of further trade in the nation. The more recent policy focus on accreditation and standardization of services would provide benefits for the entire system, if it were applied equitably. However, given the uneven nature of these measures across healthcare services, medical tourism only further dichotomizes the gaps between public and private service delivery. Without a national regulatory framework that requires the economic and infrastructural benefits of this trade to be filtered equitably across the system, problems of equity, access, quality, and cost of healthcare will only be further exacerbated.

Chapter 3

The Intersections of Tourism and Health

The Marketization of Medical Tourism

The role of "tourism" within medical tourism is often modulated or denied outright in much of the literature on the phenomenon. In this chapter, I contend that the industry and practice are both intrinsically connected to and reliant on tourism, of which is demonstrated by many of the transformations underway within the tertiary healthcare sector in Mumbai. Tourism is often mistakenly generalized as a relatively homogenous activity undertaken only for the purposes of recreation, leisure, and pleasure. However, studies of tourism from the late 1970s onwards have shown it to be a complex and highly heterogenous phenomenon, encompassing a wide range of activities, underpinned by a wide range of motivations, facilitated by an interconnected global industry. As noted by Moufakkir and Burns (2012, 1), "Tourism is a dynamic global phenomenon: an agent of change, harbinger of controversy, and a significant factor in social, cultural and technical evolution."

It was only gradually during fieldwork that the material significance and implications of medical tourism to the workings of the hospitals were progressively revealed. Very few of the people in the tertiary healthcare industry acknowledged that medical tourism had any noteworthy relevance to themselves or the hospitals where they worked. Many of my early informants were senior hospital administrators who generally avoided the topic of medical tourism, discussing instead their high-tech equipment, upgrades to their facilities, and the accreditations, awards, and accolades their respective hospitals had received. Other conversations centered on their individual or hospital's aims to guarantee that all patients could access their care, and the specific mechanisms they had in place to promote equitable delivery of care.

These voiced perspectives deftly aligned with the Indian Medical Council's (IMC) Professional Code of Ethics, which reinforce social justice values within the profession, yet masked the range and magnitude of marketing techniques oriented to medical tourism, including the sloganization of the language of hospital administrators and the varied transformations taking place in the hospitals to entice high fee-paying patients to access their services. The simultaneous promotion and denial are evident in the commodification of many goods and services but has particular valence in such a context where the state reinforces and legitimizes the dual messaging.

In the midst of the global rush toward the promotion of medical tourism, it is of significance that all of the hospitals in this research were fast to proclaim their lack of focus on medical tourism and that any flows of medical tourists into their hospitals were merely a "bi-product" of external factors: not unwelcome, but not explicitly targeted. As such, this chapter describes the agency of different actors engaging in medical tourism, from the local Trust Hospitals in the study, to international stakeholders such as multilateral institutions and multinational corporations.

There were manifold recognizable actions and transformations underway in the hospitals that corresponded with and connected to the wider tourism industry, supporting and reinforcing notions of market-led healthcare. These included the redesign and reconfiguration of physical design and infrastructure; market-led hospital branding; expansion of consumer-driven services; digital marketing of services and doctors; and partnerships with third-party facilitators. Other factors include emerging health insurance coverage and portability issues, and national marketing campaigns promoting medical tourism in India. Many of these actions and transformations are outward representations of the hypercommodified features of medical tourism. Similarly, international barriers to medical tourism also replicate that of the wider tourism industry, including macroeconomic fluctuations, political unrest, security volatility and significantly, global disease outbreaks such as that experienced amidst the international coronavirus pandemic.

As such, this chapter focuses on the means by which national efforts and those of private hospitals in Mumbai have tapped into a nascent medical tourism supply chain that has developed by attaching itself to the broader tourism supply chain. This is a mutually reinforcing relationship, which adds to the circuits of tourism production and consumption through the development and transformation of current health-related infrastructure and services.

A GLOBAL TOURISM DESTINATION

Tourism is centrally concerned with the corporeal movement of people across and within particular spatial and temporal frames. All through history people have moved across geographic spaces for any number of reasons, but contemporary forms of tourism arose alongside the more recent developments of air travel, the car industry, railways, and more regulated labor conditions. All of these factors encouraged a mass growth in the mobility of people to move back and forth across space in relatively short periods of time.

In the latter decades of the 20th century, mass tourism was the primary mode of practice, with people travelling in large groups to resort destinations such as Spain, Mexico, and the Caribbean (Marson 2011). However, mass tourism was on the decline in the late 1980s, due to the increasing popularity of niche forms of tourism and recognition of the negative impacts that arose as a consequence of the overdevelopment of favored destination locations (Robinson, Heitmann, and Dieke 2011). In little more than a century, travel for leisure and recreation has become commodified on a global scale, and travel products and markets have become far more diverse and specialized. These new niche products, including medical tourism, are marketed to people from developed and developing countries that are joining the middle class, or have become comparatively wealthy with significant disposable income to spend on leisure and recreation products.

Early tourism scholarship emerged using etic approaches to measure the economic impact of tourism. Although empirical measures remain a dominant feature of the field, qualitative approaches have emerged as new interdisciplinary subfields, using diverse methodologies, theoretical and analytical frameworks. These forms of research have led to new understandings of tourism as highly fragmented, complex and synonymous to wider international, socio-cultural processes.

One of the first major anthropological contributions to the study of tourism came via MacCannell's (1976) publication "The Tourist: A New Theory of the Leisure Class." MacCannell's primary focus was the motivations of Western tourists, who he (controversially) contended were mainly interested in seeking out authenticity in their experiences. This search for "authenticity" was conceived as a form of resistance to the expansion of modernism in the context of capitalism. From here, analysis shifted to investigations employing a dualist host–guest paradigm, with most studies focusing on the negative impact of the disempowered hosts (Chambers 1997; MacCannell 1992; Ross 1994; Yamashita, Din, and Eades 1997). Other major lines of social inquiry have formed around tourism as nonordinary behavior, and the lifecycles of specific tourism attractions.

Tourism studies have since expanded, producing a broad corpus of in-depth, critical research that expands upon earlier understandings of tourism. In particular, there has been a critique of its assumed necessary connection to "leisure and pleasure." Gale (2008, 1) argues that it moves to incorporate broader activities and practices within a tourism framework has been explained as, "in part a response to criticism of the manner in which this particular activity and the people who participate in it are defined."

However, some tourism scholars argue that social research on tourism has failed to significantly engage in critical approaches related to issues of social justice. Bianchi (2009, 484) argued that further research must focus on how tourism relates to "processes of globalization, capitalism and structural power." In doing so, he suggests that research needs to provide better understandings of the intersections of different mobilities with "global commodity chains and divisions of labor in which tourism produces and reproduces inequalities between markets and destinations, as well as amongst different categories of tourist."

Tourism has been instrumental in a range of social, cultural, and technical transformations in different contexts internationally, which, according to Moufakkir and Burns (2012), has led to its entanglement in an assortment of ongoing controversies. Some of the classic controversies involve specific forms of tourism such as thanatourism[1] and sex tourism, but also due to the negative impacts it has had on the hosts or host environment such as unsustainable tourism, overdevelopment, and exploitative employment practices.

In little more than a century, travel for leisure, recreation, and a broad spectrum of other forms, has developed into a vast and commodified global industry, with travel markets and products far more diverse and specialized than ever before. The first formal attempts to promote tourism in India occurred in the final years of British colonial rule. The British formed a tourism committee in 1945 to investigate the potential for developing the industry in the nation. The committee released a report to the Indian Government, recommending that separate tourism offices be established in Delhi, Bombay, Calcutta, and Madras to promote and develop the industry (Mishra, Rout, and Mohapatra 2011). Under the guidance of Jawaharlal Nehru, the nation's first Prime Minister, these four tourism branches were set up in 1949, alongside a national Tourist Traffic Branch, which later, in 1959, became the Department of Tourism. An additional two international offices were also established in New York and London (Seifert-Granzin and Jesupatham 1999). In 1967, the tourism industry was afforded greater national priority through its promotion to the status of Ministry of Tourism and Civil Aviation. Alongside other planning regimes in the nation, a series of five-year plans were set out to develop the sector, mainly focusing on accommodation infrastructure.

Although there were modest gains in domestic tourism during earlier decades, international tourism in India gained little traction until the neoliberal reforms of the 1990s. These reforms identified foreign tourism as a priority area for further investment with a new focus on attracting foreign arrivals. By 2002, the government's role moved from that concerned primarily with tourism regulation and infrastructure to that of marketer, creating a "global brand" strategy for the nation. It was at this time the national "Incredible

India" campaign was unveiled, aiming to shift global perceptions of India as a developing country to that of an emerging and "modern" nation.

From the mid to late 1990s, with India's steady economic growth and ongoing development of the sector, alongside the relatively stable political environment and low international exchange rate, the rate of foreign tourist arrivals accelerated, recording a fivefold increase from 1995 to 2018 (2.1 million to 10.5 million) (see figure 3.1). With the rapid increase of international tourist arrivals in the nation, the corresponding growth of foreign exchange earnings led to greater national attention on the sector. Foreign earnings rose to nearly 7% of the country's entire GDP by 2010 (see table 3.1), equivalent to half the earnings of all trade in services in India (World Bank 2014). The contribution of the tourism sector to employment in the nation is also significant, with over 12% of the nation's jobs located within the sector (see table 3.1).

With the emergence of the Covid-19 pandemic in 2020, the Indian tourism sector contracted significantly, along with that of the rest of the world.

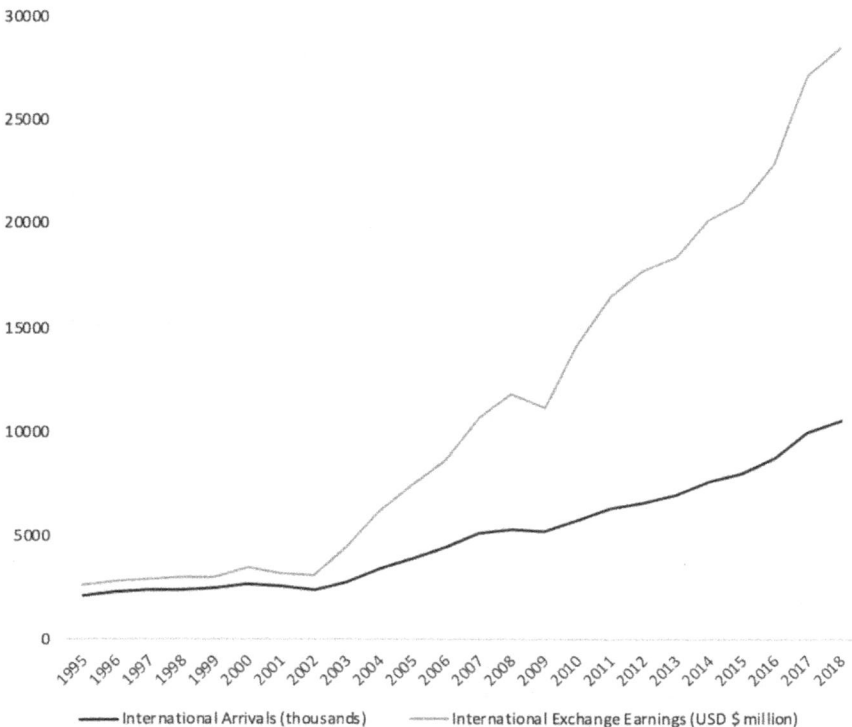

Figure 3.1   International Tourist Arrivals and Exchange Earnings in India, 1995–2018). *Source*: Government of India (2006; 2018).

Table 3.1   Contribution of Tourism to GDP and Employment

Year	GDP %	Employment %
2009–10	6.77	10.17
2010–11	6.68	10.78
2011–12	6.74	11.49
2013–14	5.68	11.37
2014–15	5.81	12.25
2015–16	5.10	12.38
2016–17	5.06	12.2
2017–18	-	12.13
2018–19	-	12.75

Sources: Government of India (2014, 70); Ministry of Tourism (2020, 96).

Global estimates of the impact in 2020 included a drop of nearly 80% of transnational tourism, equating to a loss of export revenue of about USD 1.2 trillion (UNWTO 2020). In 2019, approximately 11 million international tourists travelled to India, but in 2020 this had decreased to around three million arrivals (India Brand Equity Foundation 2021). With the coronavirus pandemic reaching crisis point in the nation in the first half of 2021, many countries globally closed their borders to anyone travelling in or out of India, signifying greater declines in international tourism arrivals. In mid-2020, the Federation of Indian Chambers of Commerce and Industry (FICCI) estimated approximately 40 million jobs and the equivalent of USD 17 billion in revenue would be lost in the following year from the Indian travel and tourism sector as a result (FICCI 2020). The long-term impacts of the coronavirus pandemic on tourism globally are still unfolding, with rolling lockdowns, border restrictions, and airline disruptions stalling and disrupting international travel. This has specific and situated implications for the future of medical tourism in India and globally as one of many forms of the broader tourism industry.

THE AFFECTIVE WORK OF BRANDING
FOR MEDICAL TOURISM

Despite mounting evidence depicting the poor outcomes of commodified healthcare for marginal groups within populations, examples of aggressive marketing of medical tourism are prevalent in India and across the globe. In 2005, the Vice President of Operations of Wockhardt Hospitals in Maharashtra was quoted in the media stating, "Branding in the healthcare sector is as important as the concept of branding in other service sectors. Consumers trust brands, similarly healthcare consumers trust healthcare brands" (Singh 2005, n.p.).

Government medical tourism brochures correlate with national tourism branding campaigns, alongside transnational finance firms (such as KPMG and Deloitte) who publish national and global reports predicting often optimistic or overstated economic projections for the sector. Medical Tourism Companies (otherwise known as medical facilitators or brokers) advertise prolifically online of the low cost and "add-on" services they provide. Somewhat provocative advertising slogans litter the Internet: "Medical Tourism. Safe. Cost-effective. And fun"; "Our mission is to contribute to a world where everybody gets access to the medical care they deserve"; "We strive to provide an affordable and delightful medical tourism experience". Browsing the virtual bookshelves of Amazon reveals a multiplicity of medical tourism "guidebooks" written in the style of Lonely Planet guides while social media is awash with self-proclaimed experts sermonizing the benefits of medical tourism for all.

The branding of a nation, a hospital, a clinic, or even a specific doctor is integral to the marketing strategies of operators within the medical tourism industry. The role of emotion, and affective work, in hospital brand building is functional and symbolic, but is also ideological. It initiates and maintains social and cultural value systems in the identity construction of both global and local healthcare consumers. Affective brand management seeks to first stimulate and appeal to consumer aspirations, emotions, and social relations, then, ultimately, commodify them.

NATIONAL BRANDING: CONSTRUCTING A SIGNATURE NICHE

Nations engaging in medical tourism often develop "signature" brands to promote and market their country, incorporating specific cultural, social, and touristic themes and markers that delineate it as a unique, niche destination. Most countries also promote specific areas or systems of medicine within their niche. For example, the Caribbean promotes medical tourism within a frame of adventure tourism, marketing indigenous herbal healing from eco-resorts situated in rainforests (Chambers and McIntosh 2008). While in Argentina, cosmetic surgery is advertised within a frame of "sensual exoticism" employing the Argentinian tango as an intrinsic cultural component of the country (Viladrich and Baron-Faust 2014).

The respective niches marketed form a nation's signature brand and are replicated across national medical tourism supply chains. The work of developing national signature tourism branding can be broadly understood as an effort to gain a comparative advantage over other countries seeking to attract medical tourists. In India, its first cohesive national tourism brand building efforts evolved via its global Incredible India campaign, launched in 2002. This campaign classified medical tourism as a subset of the broader wellness tourism industry. Promoted as a niche wellness "holiday idea, it was framed as a form of 'high-tech healing'. Marketing focused on lists of surgery and treatment options at select private hospitals across the nation, boasting 'five-star facilities' and 'world-class treatments'" (Ministry of Tourism 2006).

With some estimates as high as $4 trillion, the global wellness industry includes personal care, beauty, and antiaging; nutrition and weight loss; fitness and mind-body; preventive and personalized medicine; complementary and alternative medicine; wellness real estate; spa facilities, thermal springs; and workplace wellness. Companies internationally aggressively promote wellness, spiritual and healing retreats alongside "spa culture," particularly as a part of medical tourism packages, with "medispas."

Definitions of wellness are plural and contested, however, there are three broad categories that together capture most understandings of and approach to studies of wellness: mental state accounts, preference satisfaction, and objective lists (Caton et al. 2018, xvii–xviii). The extant literature on (health and) wellness tourism typically fall within the first, experiential, category of wellness from the standpoint of the individual tourist. However, Caton and others (2018), following Smith and Diekman (2017), note that there is a distinct gap in the literature examining host wellness "and of the ecosystem that sustains touristic activity" (Caton et al. 2018, xxi).

Although there are distinct differences in contemporary patterns and practices, India has a long history of pilgrimage for healing and death rites that are interwoven with modern modes and practices of medical tourism. Notably, the ethnographic works of Jonathon Parry (1994), Christopher Justice (1997), have detailed some of the traditional and ongoing practices of pilgrims and mourners traveling to the city of Varanasi[2] from across the world to perform specific death rites of passage. Varanasi is a major religious hub, with Hindu, Muslim, Buddhist, and Jain pilgrims making the journey to Varanasi over centuries to visit temples and shrines, and bathe in the River Ganges for curative and spiritual purposes. Varanasi's cultural heritage is diverse and extensive, with legends denoting it as the birthplace of both Shiva[3] and Parsvanatha[4], and within 10 kilometers of the site where Buddha delivered his first sermon after achieving enlightenment.

Although primarily understood within the frame of pilgrimage tourism, healing and wellness constitute key characteristics of pilgrimage to the site. For example, Barrett (2008), building on the work of Parry and Justice, has described the healing practices of the Aghori healers at Varanasi, with pilgrims most commonly seeking out Aghori medicine for infertility and a subset of dermatological disorders including leprosy and leukoderma. Aligning with national tourism trends, international tourism to Varanasi experienced significant growth in the 1990s, increasing four-fold from 284,000 in 1991 to 1,238 million in 2000 (Singh and Rana 2001).

Another early development associated to wellness tourism was the establishment of hill station retreats by the British raj. Hill stations, indicative of the name, are located in places of higher elevation and were founded for broadly therapeutic purposes, as places of respite and recuperation. During colonial rule, the British often escaped the tropical[5] heat and pollution of the towns and cities by retreating to popular hill stations in Darjeeling, Kashmir, Shimla, and Ooty, most of which were established in the mid-19th century (Connell 2016). At many hill stations, the British set out to recreate environments similar to those of England, experimenting with the growing of fruits, flowers, and vegetables found "at home" and artificially creating lakes similar the English countryside. Bhattacharya (2013) has contended that these transformations of the landscape by the British constituted a distinctive form of colonial urbanism.

The hills of Darjeeling were of particular interest to the East India Company, wresting the district from the Raja of Sikkim in the late 1830s, with the prospect of building a sanatorium in the area. In a letter to the Raja in 1835 pursuing occupation of the land, an officer of the Governor General wrote that it was to be used "for the purpose of enabling the servants of his government, suffering from the sickness, to avail themselves of its advantages" (Kumari 2017). The subsequent construction of Eden sanatorium, multiple hotels, and at least 70 European style houses by the early 1850s led to the hill station's popularity as a colonial outpost, of medicalized leisure and influential British colonists and Indian elites alike, as a summer retreat across the 19th century and early decades of the 20th century (Mukherjee 2010).

In the 1960s, the recuperative features of hill stations such as Darjeeling, and spiritual heritage of places like Varanasi, started attracting international tourists seeking spiritual and wellness alternatives, particularly those offered by Indian traditional medicine, such as yoga and meditation (Laing and Weiler 2008). In the late 1960s, advocates of India's meditation and yoga teachings included high profile Western celebrities, including members of The Beatles and The Rolling Stones, further cultivating India's reputation as a global spiritual hub (Telej and Gamble 2019).

These early examples of wellness tourism were the precursor to an expanding and highly commodified "wellness" tourism industry across the nation. Indian wellness tourism, the banner under which medical tourism is classified, includes the mass production and sale of ayurvedic herbal medicines and remedies by pharmaceutical companies. FDI India, a network of foreign investment facilitators, has reported that India is the second largest exporter of ayurvedic and alternative medicine internationally (FDI India 2021).

The promotion of medical tourism through national and global platforms, such as the Incredible India campaign, serves a variety of both economic and political purposes. Of particular interest is the state-led promotion of the private tertiary healthcare. Ong (2010) has described the connections of the affective work of promoting biotechnologies in Asia, where they are associated with "nationalist efforts to overcome past humiliations and to restore national identity" and a "deep nationalist fervor in the race to be "number one" in cutting-edge sciences, with its promise of a lucrative science-driven economy" (Ong 2010, 3). She argues that this helps to legitimize state investment and promotion of biotechnologies. Similar processes are at play here, promoting the "world-class" facilities and services provided by the private tertiary healthcare sector (see chapters 3 and 5 for further detail).

Hospitals and health professionals engaging in the trade are highly dependent on the Indian government for the marketing of medical tourism. Dr Lulla, for example, contended it should be the Indian government's responsibility to promote medical tourism, as this would prevent patients from suspecting the economic intent motivating individual providers or their hospitals. Dr Lulla noted, "[T]here are many factors, but I think the breaking line will be how India markets itself, because I can't market the hospital individually. It will be obvious that, yes, I'm marketing because I want more patients." Dr Lulla described this as a paradox for hospitals and health professionals alike, as their primary intent should be to offer quality care to patients, yet this is all too often subverted by the need to attract high-fee-paying patients to maintain economic viability (see chapter 4 for more detail).

While hospitals and health workers aspire for greater engagement and support from government, public health advocates across India have been vocal in their criticism of the government's promotion of the medical tourism industry. For instance, Duggal (2007) and Reddy and Qadeer (2012) have both argued that given the state of the ailing public health system, any government connection to medical tourism is grossly unethical. Further, Duggal contends that any fiscal incentives and subsidies directed to large participating hospitals should be conditional, and that the idle capacity of these hospitals should be formally required to provide free care for Indian residents who do not have the means to pay.

The Indian Government has paid little heed to such critiques, providing significant direct and "soft" promotion and incentives for the sector through a range of policy and legislative levers from the early 2000s. The 2002 National Health Policy (NHP) contained early example of the Indian government's promotion of medical tourism. The NHP addressed the provision of "medical facilities to users from overseas," declaring treatment of international patients as an "export," with those providing medical tourism services deemed "eligible for all fiscal incentives extended to export earnings" (Directorate-General of Health Services 2002).

Another mechanism introduced in 2005 by the Indian government to facilitate medical tourism was the supposedly fast-tracked medical visa category, introduced to minimize processing and bureaucratic interventions that may hinder or impede potential medical tourists from gaining access to services in the country. The medical visa is valid for up to 12 months, facilitating multiple entries to the country. It also allows two family members of the visa holder to be granted "attendant" visas with the same conditions applied. However, some in the industry have claimed that cumbersome requirements of the medical visa have, in fact, made it more difficult for medical tourists to gain entry to the country for care ('Stricter visa rules driving away medical tourism from India' 2013).

TOURISM IMAGINARIES AND THE CONSTRUCTION OF "HOSPITELS"

It became evident during fieldwork that the hospitals of focus all initiated a range of other changes and engaged in practices aligned with the tourism market, designed to attract medical tourists. The physical attributes of the hospitals attracting higher numbers of medical tourists were visibly different to other hospitals. These hospitals could easily be mistaken for the many international luxury hotels located in Mumbai. Both the external and internal physical design of hospitals in India are transforming in a manner that mirror and replicate the luxury hotel industry in India. The proliferation of luxury hotels across the nation was noted in Forbes magazine, stating that "the country, once a cheap travel destination and long associated with poverty and strife, is now becoming famous for its luxury hotels" (Le Draoulec 2007). The palatial architecture used by the Oberoi, Leila, and Taj luxury hotel chains are uncannily similar to many of the high-end private tertiary hospitals emerging in the city, so much so that it can be difficult to distinguish between them. The use of architecture to signal wealth and conspicuous consumption has a lengthy history that is expressed in diverse forms across different contextual urban landscapes. Large-scale architectural design, including temples, palaces, and royal tombs have symbolized and reinforced power structures in social organization for centuries (Reigel 2020).

The parallels of this new class of private, prestigious hospitals offering health services for medical travelers (and elite nationals), with the luxury five-star hotel industry do not arise by coincidence. It is a carefully crafted representation that uses architecture as a language to evoke specific Orientalist imaginaries of India and, seemingly paradoxically, the modernism of its private healthcare institutions. The evident tension between these two ostensibly juxtaposed metanarratives—a past seductive opulence of the maharajas and their grand palaces, alongside cutting-edge, global biotechnical futures of radical innovation—must be understood within the broader frames of both commodification and globalization and a wider historicity, embedded across the chain of tourism production.

The concept of tourism imaginaries emerged from understandings of social imaginaries, articulated by Appadurai (1996) as the collective social practice of imagination. Salazar's (2012) framing of tourism imaginaries and their diffusion encourages us to think about where imaginaries of people and places originate, and how "lived spaces are shaped by and are shaping tourism practices and fantasies." (Salazar 2012, 3). In particular, Salazar focuses on the production of tourism imaginaries of "otherness" and how these imaginaries are negotiated, circulated, and perpetuated globally. In Salazar and Graburn's edited collection "Tourism Imaginaries: Anthropological Approaches" (2014), the authors outline a series of place-based examples to inform critical anthropological frameworks focusing on the complex origins, global circulation, and implications of tourism imaginaries on lived experiences for both tourists and hosts.

The palatial architecture, used first by the five-star hotels of India followed by the large private hospitals attracting medical tourists, (re)produce tourist imaginaries of luxurious colonial palaces of high imperialism of Britain, aligning with oriental, colonial, and imperial discourses of the past, of which Salazar (2012, 9) notes are often "fertile ground for nostalgic and romantic dreams." Other anthropological works on tourism imaginaries have focused on self–other relations; the notion that people travel not only to experience otherness and alterity, but also to play out fantasies of the "other in us" (Pandian and Parman 2004; Graburn 2012; Picard and Di Giovine 2014). Discourses of traveling from afar for medical treatment in a hospital evocative of a grand palace such as the Taj Mahal, speaks to more than engaging in imaginaries of India, but also of playing out fantasies of British colonial decadence, or the Shah's decadence, in one's own life. For wellness-focused tourism, especially when sick, these self–other relations would potentially hold even greater importance.

There are further ways we can understand hospitals' replication of the architecture and design of five-star luxury hotels. First, in the way it supports their normative insertion to wider cultural circuits of global tourism production and supply. Bochaton and Lefebvre's (2009) work on the heterotopic spaces created by hospitals attracting medical tourism in India and Thailand engages with some of these processual transitions underway in the sector. They posit that hospitals "are being rethought through this prism of medical tourism" and that in their recreation, "hospitals face a dilemma of trying to

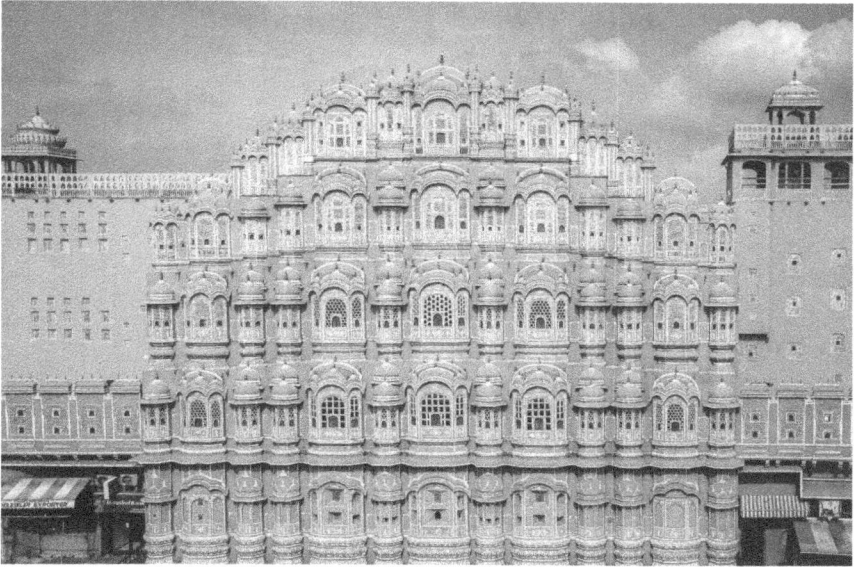

Figure 3.2   Hawa Mahal Palace in Jaipur. *Source*: De Dishari (2021). Architecture/
Buildings. Pixabay.

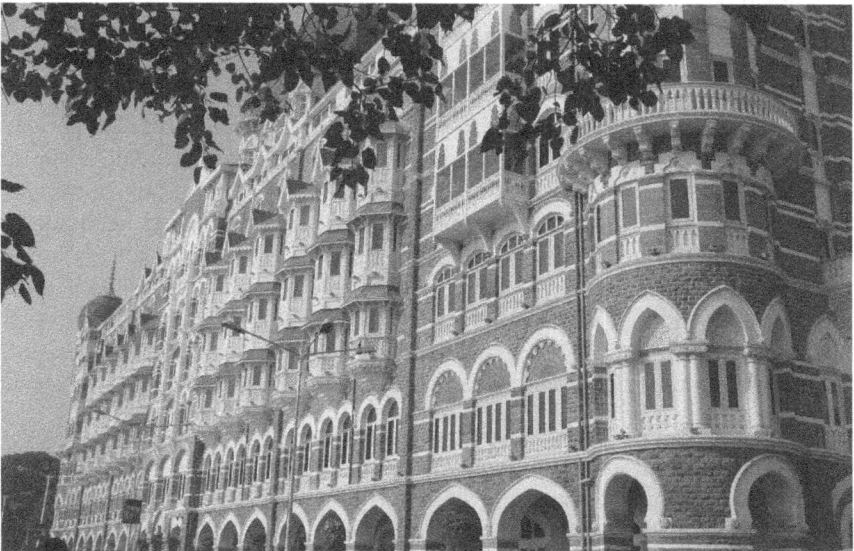

Figure 3.3   The Taj Hotel in Mumbai. *Source*: Ramkrishna (2021). Image of Nature.
Pixabay.

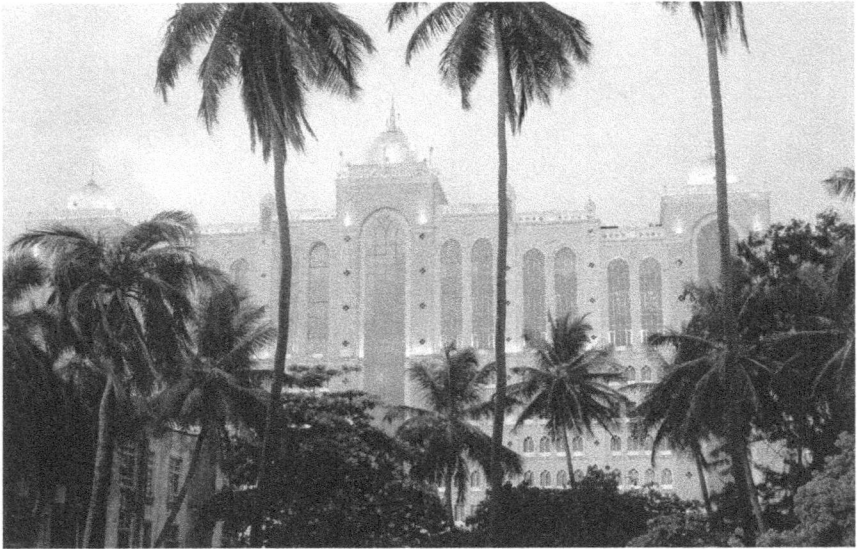

Figure 3.4   Private Hospital in Hyderabad. *Source*: Ramkrishna (2021).Tech Gurug. Pixabay.

meet local healthcare needs as well as the expectations of a tourism industry standard" (2009, 91).

Other studies focusing on dedicated medical or healthcare hotels have highlighted how internal architectural and spatial design replicate the benefits, convenience, and comfort provided by hotels, not usually provided by hospitals, and can positively influence medical tourists' choices in site selection (Han et al. 2015; Illing 2016). Such facilities could include lavish entrance lobbies, gymnasiums, swimming pools, suites accommodating accompanying carers, and dining facilities. In particular, the two newer hospitals in this study, Ramrakhyani and Tayyib, are impressively lavish buildings, both inside and out. The hospitals also purported to conform to, or exceed, the physical attributes of "world-class" hospital standards. For example, when discussing the inflow of medical tourism at Ramrakhyani Hospital, Dr Lulla explained:

> We have won a lot of international accolades. The hospital is not less than any other international hospital in terms of quality and infrastructure that we provide. We have our bed space ratio of one to 1,600 square feet, which is much larger than American standards provide. We have state of the art equipment, air conditioning systems, infection control protocols, trained nursing staff and international faculty. So, we have the best in services and infrastructure.

Many hospitals in India vying to attract medical tourists offer a range of premium accommodation suites. All hospitals in the study had between five and seven different "classes" of rooms. As noted earlier, several of the hospitals where I undertook my fieldwork offer luxury "suites," usually located on the top floor of the multistorey institutions. These suites come with surround sound music systems, modern wide-screen televisions with cable access, personal attendants, extra guest bedrooms, kitchenettes, fully fitted out bathrooms, computer facilities with internet, and pick-up and drop-off services in luxury cars. The room fees for these high-end rooms also mirror the rates for luxury hotels. Ramrakhyani Hospital offered one such suite for approximately USD 450 per night, which did not include medical fees. The suites in private hospitals are also often named the "Presidential Suite," which is also how the best rooms at the luxury hotel chains across the nation are referred to.

All but one of the hospitals in the study were in the process of creating a range of "value adding" services for medical tourists. The international client manager at one of the hospitals explained that they were adding a range of different services to encourage medical tourism, such as setting up an international counter in the lobby to assist international patients. She noted that the international counter would be a "one-stop-shop" that could arrange phone and internet plans, diet preferences and alongside the other medical aspects of their treatment.

The tasks that were to be carried out by the "international counter" parallel that of a hotel's concierge. Other hospital concierge services that were either in place or in the process of implementation at the hospitals included arranging: airport transfers for patients (with luxury European cars), specific tailored meals for patients and people traveling with them, references to Ayurvedic practitioners (often associated with the hospital), and researching and booking post-procedure travel arrangements. An ophthalmologist explained how these services impact on the price of surgery packages offered through the hospital, "most cataract surgeries are day care packages; you operate in the morning and within a few hours the patient is discharged. But a patient may want to be staying in a special room or a suite. Now here we have medical tourists who is coming down and the cataract charges could be increased, because he's availing of the facilities."

Three of the hospitals in the study had international package deals for a range of "treatments" such as cardiac procedures, orthopedic and joint replacement, human reproduction procedures, bariatric surgery, aesthetic/cosmetic procedures, dental services, gynecology, ophthalmology, general surgery, and ENT surgery. Of these hospitals, only one had significantly different pricing scales for international patients comparatively to local patients, where they added an extra 25% to the cost of the treatment. However, they all had a sliding scale of accommodation, with the most expensive, high-end rooms and suites promoted as the primary option for medical tourists. Khalsa Hospital also had partnerships with multiple high-end hotels that are located within close proximity, where patients or their accompanying carers were able access the rooms at a reduced rate. These pricing strategies and associated structures linking to the elite end of the broader tourism industry illustrate that the hospitals were well aware they were servicing patients at the top stratum of a dual-tier system, and that there is a substantial difference between a local and medical tourist's capacity to pay.

THE AFFECTIVE BRANDING OF
HOSPITAL SITES AND SPACES

Beyond that of the affective architecture, hospitals are also engaging in other affective practices such as affective signature spatial branding, with strategies aligning with other highly commodified goods and services. For example, Carl Jon Way Ng (2019) has described the branded space of McDonalds stores, which "stimulate wholesome fun and pleasure with its semiotics of brightly coloured décor and uniforms, Disney toys and Happy Meals, among other things, and hence the consumer's socio-affective connection with the brand" (Ng 2019, 126). All hospitals in the study used marketing slogans to build their brand. Some used religious tagging: "When I fall sick it is HE who cures me." Others incorporated AYUSH services, promoting a wellbeing approach, such as "Harmonious Health and Healing." This form of branding forms part of the affective work used to build the trust of health consumers and validate the ventures in the broader state healthcare system (Ong 2016).

The website of Khalsa Hospital used a variety of promotional factors. As you enter the website, elevator-style music automatically plays on repeat, while the animated site loads, espousing the family values imbued in the hospital and staff. In another section of the website, under the tag of "Medical Tourism," a header reads "Using Technology with Tender Loving Care," emphasizing the "sophisticated technology," "medical brilliance," and "personalized care" on offer. This idea that each hospital creates an environment of familial care was a feature promoted by three of the hospitals under study. Further, all five hospitals associated their branding with the idea of technologically advanced biomedicine.

In discussion with one of the Management staff at Ramrakhyani Hospital, he explained what he saw as the most important element for his hospital to increase medical tourism over time. He identified three factors that enhance a hospital's international reputation: appropriate accreditation; low comparative cost of services; and, what he called the "happiness factor." On further enquiry, he explained the "happiness factor" as the satisfaction of patients with their overall experience of the hospital. He went on to state that a "leading independent company" had conducted a survey of hospitals, finding their hospital had the fifth highest "happiness" rating in the country. Many hospital administrators and medical staff had sloganized their language, sometimes subtly, or perhaps inadvertently, but in other cases it was most certainly a practiced and polished performance of affective labor.

The hospital's online presence further supported this "happiness factor" in a hyperbolic affective framework of wellness, stating,

> We have become the physical face of a new generation. We have become the collective psyche of a vibrant India's energy, drive and vitality. We have become the language of new passion, of affluence, of happiness that begins with an individual, and culminates into the wellbeing of an entire society.

Other more surprising methods used by hospitals applying affective branding techniques also came to light during fieldwork. Before leaving Australia, the discussions I had with friends, family, and colleagues who had been to India before invariably broached the subject of the overwhelming, unfamiliar, and generally unpleasant smells they associated with the country. Whether their associations were linked to that of incense, pungent spices, or excrement, the memory of these aromas loomed large in the memories they shared. In my case, the smell of anise now instantaneously takes me to the kitchen of my Hindi teacher, who taught me how to cook a particular dish using the spice. Or how the smell of *chai* transports me to overcrowded sleeper trains, rumbling through the night with constant processions of *chai-wallahs* selling their goods, with their booming chants of *garam chaaaaiiiiiiii, garam chaaaaiiiiiiii*. These are not vague memories that come to mind, but those of fine detail. Consumer research has examined the effect of scents when marketing products and has shown a positive correlation between ambient scents and consumption practices (Canniford, Riach, and Hill 2018). Although I did not recognize it at the time, one of the hospitals in this study marketed and characterized their "consumer" experience through the use of aroma.

One afternoon, I was sitting in one of the large, light-filled ground-floor waiting rooms of Ramrakhyani Hospital, waiting to interview a general manager of the hospital. The waiting room had multiple consultancy suites situated around the space, with seating for over 50 people spread sparsely across the area. In the middle of the waiting room was an oval reception bench, with two crisply uniformed and highly groomed female staff members. I had been waiting to see the manager for nearly two hours when my attention was drawn to a busy hospital attendant across the other side of the room. What specifically caught my eye was his equipment and the task he was performing. Strapped to his back he wore what, on first examination, appeared to be a garden weed-killer backpack, spray hose attachment included. He moved slowly around the room, spraying the floor and around the waiting room chairs with this device.

Although I had spent several elongated periods of time in this waiting room over preceding months observing the general comings and goings, this was unfamiliar. My curiosity peaked, first wondering why it was that this up-market, temperature-controlled, sparkling clean hospital was protecting itself against weeds growing within its midst. At the time, the city was in the midst of the 2009 swine influenza epidemic, making my second guess that it was some type of sanitization equipment designed to allay the fears of patients regarding the "safety" of the environment through a visual display. As the man slowly, methodically, wove his way closer to me, I was able to get a closer look at his equipment.

This provided no further clues, as there was no branding, or other obvious pointers on the backpack or spraying attachment. It was only when the attendant was within approximately a meter of me that I detected a pleasant floral aroma wafting across the room, which is when it struck me. The hospital attendant wasn't attempting to kill indoor weeds. He wasn't putting on a show of the sanitary measures in place; he was perfuming the room. As I continued with my observations and interviews in the hospital, I was regularly told of how much different this hospital was to other institutions. Hospital workers would exclaim, "Don't you feel more at home here? It doesn't even smell like a hospital!"

Although the physical attributes of the hospitals were viewed as an impor-tant factor for attracting international patients, doctors and hospital man-agement personnel would recite the numerous features of their respective hospitals that they believed would be attractive to foreign patients, building their brand. One doctor explained:

> We need to give quality service provision...the rooms have to be good. the ambi-
> ence has to be good. then the approach to patients has to be good. You have
> to make them feel at home because they are leaving their country and they are
> coming here. So, you have to give them something that is better than what they
> are experiencing within their country.

Differentiation between how these new attributes and functions are pro-moted is the point of departure in the private tertiary sector. The corporate, for-profit hospitals generally employ far more outward and aggressive mar-keting tactics than the Trust hospitals, who incorporated an understated style during the transformation of their brand. Dr Rao explained the approach of Ramrakhyani Hospital:

> I will keep on doing my genuine work. If I'm doing research, I'll publish it. If
> my doctor is doing something good, he will publish his general article. If people

are concerned about quality, when they do a search, they'll come to know what good work that person has done. So that is what we do, but we don't overtly market ourselves outside this country. That is not our focus. Because then, people will really feel that you're doing it for getting patients.

Dr Rao's explanation of the quasi-marketing strategies used by hospitals to build their brand, and Dr Lulla's admission that they don't want to noticeably promote to medical tourists reveals the fine line trod by many private Trust Hospitals in India. The concession that they will unobtrusively promote features that they understand are marketable infers a deeper level of consideration. This speaks to multiple issues, including the problems of overtly offering market-led services in a not-for-profit environment and the professional and ethical dilemmas posed for health professionals in this context. As such, why are Trust hospitals engaging in medical tourism at all? The answer is inextricably linked to the progressively precarious economic position of Trust hospitals within the tertiary healthcare market, and the steps they are taking to remain financially viable, which is outlined in greater detail in chapter 4.

HOSPITAL ACCREDITATION AS QUALITY BRANDING

Another key strategy relied on by hospitals to promote their services to medical tourists is via hospital accreditation. Hospital accreditations have been touted internationally as a means to confirm quality and safety of services, particularly in developing countries. Hospital accreditations have also become one of the most effective marketing strategies used by hospitals in India to promote themselves to international patients and to justify claims of equivalent international standards commonly advertised by India's medical tourism sector. Dr Lulla explained why India's National Accreditation Board for Hospitals and Healthcare Providers (NABH) was developed:

It's the perception of this country being very poor; that the infrastructure, the culture and the quality of healthcare is not good. The processes have already been started by Quality Council of India coming in the picture [with] the NABH and getting recognized by ISQua. They are trying to say they are as good as any international standards. So, this hospital is accredited, that means the quality is good. You can come now and not worry about anything happening outside the hospital.

In an interview with the Manager of Admissions and Billing at Tayyib Hospital, Ms. Chatterjee, I questioned her about whether she thought that accreditations were important for hospitals in attracting foreign patients. She explained, "Yes, it is 100% important. It is a branded international marketing tool. Corporate sectors are adapting for this very reason." Ms. Chatterjee further posited that corporate hospitals were extremely strong lobbyists as they had been instrumental in the creation of the NABH. She also explained how the elite hospitals in the private sector had moved quickly to attain international accreditations that were perceived as more relevant to patients from the countries they wanted to attract.

Accreditations are also used to attract third-party facilitators such as MTCs, insurers, local and international governments, making them an important part of the medical tourism supply chain network. Dr Desai explained how one of the hospitals used their NABH accreditation to provide an advantage when creating alliances with medical insurance companies, noting "medical insurance companies will not grant insurance for patients who want to get operated on in hospitals that are not accredited."

The level and type of accreditation is important for hospitals, often dependent on the prestige and esteem attached to the organizations that sponsor or undertake the accreditation. India had several different bodies that awarded accreditations, the most prestigious offered through the NABH. The Government of India and the Confederation of Indian Industry (CII) partnered to initiate the NABH through the Quality Council of India (QCI). QCI is a non-profit society that consists of six accreditation councils. Application and annual membership fees apply for medical bodies accredited under this system. Although this local body is responsible for the NABH, it forms part of an international network of evaluators, the International Society for Quality in Healthcare (ISQua). ISQua has partners in 200 countries globally and provides accreditation for national accreditors that are members of its network.

The NABH accreditation was highly sought after by hospitals in the private sector, particularly in the urban cities of the nation. During fieldwork, there were already 324 hospitals that had been awarded an NABH and was increasingly viewed as necessary to maintain competitiveness with other hospitals. When questioning the Financial Director of Sacred Heart Hospital, Mr Rodriguez, about why Indian hospitals were so eager to attain NABH accreditation, he explained "everybody knows that unless you are certain to excel and be more than in line with the competition...I mean, it's like a force of circumstances rather than anything else." In Mumbai alone, there were 13 hospitals that had been awarded the NABH accreditation, including Sacred Heart, Khalsa, Tayyib, and Ramrakhyani hospitals.

Many of the larger private, corporate hospitals also sought out specific international accreditations. Joint Commission International (JCI), which functions as a division of The Joint Commission (TJC), was the most coveted accreditation by hospitals wanting to increase their inflow of medical tourism.

Dr Lulla explained how different accreditations were used to brand hospitals as a tool to attract patients.

> JCI is branding. There are many hospitals in the world who are not accredited but are good. [If] I'm a layman, I'm a patient, I want to know. I may read Quality Council of India's article and see whether this hospital is accredited, and it is good. Yes, so that label is important.

Although the Joint Commission is a not-for-profit organization, in 2013, the average cost of attaining a full hospital JCI accreditation was USD 52,000 (Joint Commission International 2015). However, this fee represents only a small portion of the cost of meeting the standards, excluding the outlay needed to bring a hospital in alignment with the prescribed standards. Many hospitals during fieldwork did not even have the basic information technology systems in place to record, monitor, and demonstrate to an accrediting body their history of quality and safety in clinical areas.

The high costs of attaining accreditation immediately privilege hospitals in nations with stronger macroeconomies and larger hospitals with greater financial backing, such as the corporate healthcare conglomerates in India. In 2021, there were 36 hospitals in India that had received the JCI hospital accreditation, of which 10 were located in Maharashtra (see table 3.2), all being corporate hospitals.

As a panelist for a public forum at held the University of Melbourne in 2012, entitled "Nip & Tuck, Treatment & Transplant: Medical Tourism in

Table 3.2 International Accreditations in Medical Tourism Destinations

Country	JCI Accreditations—Hospital Care	ISQua-Associated Accreditation Organizations (Hospital Related)
Cuba	-	-
Costa Rica	2	-
Mexico	6	-
Jordan	8	Health Care Accreditation Council
United Arab Emirates	196	-
Singapore	5	-
Thailand	59	The Healthcare Accreditation Institute (Public Organization)
Malaysia	17	Malaysian Society for Quality in Health
India	36	National Accreditation Board for Hospitals and Healthcare Providers

Source: International Society for Quality in Health Care (2015); Joint Commission International (2021).

Table 3.3   Accreditations of Hospitals in Study

Hospital	JCI	NABH	ISO	Other Related
A	X	✓	X	X
Sacred Heart	X	✓	Pathological laboratory Blood bank Imaging Department	X
Khalsa	X	✓	X	X

Tayyib	X	✓	Pharmacy
			Physiotherapy and
			  Rehabilitation
			Front office
			CSSD
			CAM
			Purchase
			Human Resource
			  Department
				NABL Laboratories

Ramrakhyani	X	✓	✓	X

Source: Fieldnotes (2021).

Asia," I asked the director of a major MTC based in Thailand, why her company places such an emphasis on partnering with hospitals with JCI accreditations. She explained that it was central facet of the company's ethical approach, where this vetting process protected and reassured her Australian client base that they would receive healthcare of an "international standard."

Another form of accreditation branding that has emerged as a subset of medical tourism is that of Halal accreditations for hospitals and other medical products and services, marketing accredited healthcare to Muslim medical tourists. Halal accreditations certify that a hospital complies with Halal standards. In 2012, Global Health City, a hospital in Chennai, was the first medical service in India to attain halal accreditation. In a study of the Halal accreditation of the Global Health City Hospital, Medhekar and Haq (2019) argued that halal accreditations are a signature form of affective medical tourism branding, as well as a subset of spiritual tourism branding.

AFFECTIVE DIGITAL MARKETING

Digital advertising for medical tourism has expanded over past years, often driven by MTCs, but increasingly the hospitals engaging in medical tourism are also using these tools to advertise their services to international patients. Often websites promoting medical tourism accentuate issues including the uniqueness of place (Holliday et al. 2015), whiteness (Viladrich and Baron-Faust 2013), alongside the quality of care and honesty of the providers (Guiry

2010; Lunt et al. 2014). Viladrich and Baron Faust (2013) have emphasized the growth of this form of advertising as reinforcing the commercialization of healthcare services, in its direct positioning of potential patients as consumers.

At the time of fieldwork, three of the five hospitals in the study had developed their own websites with sections focusing on medical tourists. In the following years, the remaining two hospitals also developed their own websites. The websites employed various affective tools to advertise their services. Some of the primary details on these sites include patient testimonials; video footage of the hospital and staff and/or virtual tours; photo galleries of the hospital; details of surgery and travel "packages," including pricing schedules; doctor and specialist profiles; and medical publications that outline their staff's research and development. Most hospital websites also have international patient testimonials indicating the appeal of this form of marketing to an audience seeking assurance of quality care. Several examples below demonstrate the usual form and tone of these testimonials:

After intensive Internet research I decided in November to come to India for health. From the outset they were efficient & informative & answered in writing all of my questions. I cannot praise enough the efficiency of the hospital from the initial consultation with Dr [X], the testing procedures & then finally the procedures themselves. It could not have been more comprehensive. Though I cannot see the final result, I am confident that the outcome will be excellent. I would recommend this facility & Dr [X] without reservation.

(United Kingdom patient testimonial)

My experience at [this] Hospital has been very wonderful in view of the excellent professional service I received from Dr [X] who was directly assigned to handle my case like Diabetes, Parkinson & High blood pressure. The PRO in person [X] has been particularly friendly and committed in her relationship with us. On a general note, the nurses the kitchen staff and housekeepers have been punctual, diligent & effective in the performance of their duties. [This] Hospital is a world class health establishment that remains a problem solver now in the future. I recommend the hospital without hesitation to all those that may be in need of its services.

(Nigerian patient testimonial)

Both examples are indicative of the types of elements the hospitals wish to highlight to potential tourists. First, that the medical tourist recommends the hospital's doctors, testing regimes, and outcomes, and that the services they received were efficient and effective as a form of assurance for prospective patients.

PARTNERSHIPS WITH THIRD-PARTY FACILITATORS

As noted, the reluctance of not-for-profit hospitals to directly advertise for foreign patients indicates their high reliance on third-party facilitators to attract medical tourists. Although many doctors regarded word-of-mouth as one of the most useful tools in attracting medical tourists, it does not readily facilitate rapid expansion of that component of their revenue stream or service delivery. It is through these third-party facilitators that the hospitals' engagement with the medical tourism supply chain is most visible. MTCs, or medical tourism brokers, are run as niche travel agencies specializing in medical tourism. These companies have proliferated internationally, "facilitating" the travel of patients to their medical "destinations." Each of the hospitals in this study had formal connections with various brokers, ranging from 2 to 15 MTCs, depending on the hospital. Although group package deals are a common marketing strategy for tourism agencies, using the same strategies to advertise surgical procedures is indicative of the hypercommodification that has emerged globally in healthcare service provision.

MTCs promoting medical tourism in India typically highlight and promote the "tourism" element strongly by attaching traditional tourist packages to medical trips. Common advertising techniques will promote pre- or postoperative trips to some of India's well-known tourist destinations, such as trips to the "golden triangle," "jungle safaris," or wellness-oriented "beachside recoveries on the golden sands of Goa." Aside from bringing patients to hospital partners, another benefit for hospitals is the outsourcing of management of any additional nonmedical needs of the international patients.

Although MTCs alleviate some of the nonmedical aspects of medical tourism, Dr Lulla explained that it was not his hospital's preferred pathway for attracting medical tourists, as MTCs charge fees to the hospital, "depending on the medical tourist, they will charge a certain percentage. We don't charge excess to the patient, but. I may have to pay a small fee to the medical tourist company. It would be more expensive for me to take a medical tourist." Despite these additional fees charged, the partnerships between MTCs and the hospitals have expanded. In 2013, Thomas Cook India, a well-known travel agency, opened an outlet branch within Khalsa hospital, under the hospital's "shop-in-shop" model, focusing on strategically aligned retail expansion.

As noted earlier, doctors and hospital administrators were quick to contest their commercial or professional interest in medical tourism as a general rule. However, an obvious question emerges from their attachment to MTCs: if the hospitals have no interest in attracting medical tourism, why do they engage in such arrangements? Further, there are specific sections of the Indian Medical Council's (Professional Conduct, Etiquette, and Ethics) Regulations (2002, 6.1.1) explicitly noting that "Soliciting of patients directly or indirectly, by a physician, by a group of physicians or by institutions or organisations is unethical." This is further reinforced by section 7.19, "A Physician shall not use touts or agents for procuring patients." So then, what of the MoU's with agents soliciting and procuring international patients, signed by all hospitals in this study, and many of the larger private hospitals across the nation?

THE IMPACT OF MULTISCALED DISRUPTIVE "EVENTS" FOR DESTINATION COUNTRIES

Disruptive events at local, national, and/or international levels can have a significant impact on the spatial direction and level of medical tourism, similar to other global trends of tourism. These events can be differentiated from general drivers of medical tourism, such as home country healthcare system deficiencies, by their rapid emergence and capacity to immediately shift medical tourism flows. I categorize the events that influence the flows of medical tourism to specific nation's most significantly driven by sudden macroeconomic fluctuations; political unrest and security volatility; and disease outbreaks. These events have a similar impact across the entire spectrum of the tourism sector, redirecting people toward or away from particular destinations.

Regardless of the use of branding, there are multiple internal and external factors that impact on the medical tourism flows into host nations, many of which cannot be directly managed or controlled by the Indian government or the wider industry. One of the perceived barriers to medical tourism raised by multiple informants was what they saw as the national lack of cultural engagement with tourism and hospitality services. To change the "attitude" or culture of tourism, several fiercely contended that it was the responsibility of the government to prioritize tourism as a sector, creating education campaigns about "hospitality" for international tourism. For example, Dr Lulla explained that India has not had a national focus on international tourism in the same manner as countries such as Thailand or Singapore, where, "their bread and butter are tourism, okay, so everything revolves around tourism. So, their cultural approach and receiving a guest, everything boils down to hard-core courtesy and tourism aspects, which is not there in India."

The lack of portability of medical insurance in many countries was another factor that was viewed by many senior hospital administrators as limiting the growth of medical tourism in Indian. This directly links with the issue of quality and safety accreditation, where the drive for accreditation from the service providers originates from two main concerns. The first relates to the expectation of an international patient who wants assurances that the quality and safety of the services being offered are at a similar standard to that offered in their own country. The second, central to the concerns of providers, is to fulfill the expectations of medical insurance companies overseas in order to facilitate access to potential patients. This concern is also pertinent due to the GATS negotiations covering insurance services, as the current offers from developed countries do not include insurance as part of the agreement. However, as early as 2007, some large health insurance corporations allowed for reimbursements to patients for treatments "outsourced" in external nations. For example, in the United States, Blue Cross and Blue Shield have provisions for patients to access treatments in particular institutions in India, as do BUPA for patients from the United Kingdom (Terry 2007).

Other developments in the type of health insurance policies offered to patients internationally include what is labeled "satellite insurance" for diasporic populations, where the majority of health services covered must be accessed in the person's country of origin. For example, Planet Hospital offers a satellite insurance policy for El Salvadorians residing in the United States, providing a cap on doctors' visits, pharmaceuticals, and emergency care that can be accessed within the country. All other care must be undertaken back in El Salvador with a doctor in their network. Unlike many policies that have exceptionally high deductibles over and above that covered by the policy, this policy covers all costs apart from travel and accommodation. In 2015, the policy was USD 200 per month for a four-person family, compared to a standard American policy, which was upward of USD 1,000 (Joint Commission International 2011; National Accreditation Board for Hospitals and Healthcare Providers 2015).

BUPA have also moved into the global medical tourism market, offering "global health plans." These policies provide coverage for medical treatments in over 800,000 hospitals internationally, including 38 hospitals in India. Ramrakhyani Hospital is one of BUPA's providers in Mumbai. BUPA also offer a short-term, 3- to 11-month global plan that covers their customers for treatments of up to USD 1.7 million. As insurance policies internationally become more flexible, the barriers to medical tourism will decrease. However, it is also likely to consolidate the market for particular corporate tertiary healthcare conglomerates that have greater access to flows of capital and technology to attain the accreditations required for international insurance affiliations.

SUDDEN MACROECONOMIC FLUCTUATIONS

Given that one of the most highly cited factors of medical tourists choosing a destination country is the price of the medical service sought, it is of no surprise that fluctuations within the international finance system can lead to conditions that make particular nations more or less favorable for medical tourists. For example, the Asian financial crisis of the late 1990s is widely cited as one of the major factors shifting the direction and flow of medical tourism across the globe. After the crash, many of the emerging Asian middle classes were no longer in the financial position to access the private tertiary healthcare system that had expanded exponentially in the previous decades. As such, private providers sought to broaden their market base to foreign patients. In the context of the devalued currencies, prices for medical and healthcare services had dropped significantly, making the proposition more favorable for overseas patients (Connell 2011). Similar upturns or downturns in the international finance system have significant potential to shape the flow of medical tourism. Macroeconomic fluctuations at the international level similarly impact on levels of international tourism. During the 2008 GFC, international tourism dropped 8% in the first quarter of the year, in the first significant downturn for decades.

POLITICAL UNREST AND SECURITY VOLATILITY

The level of political cohesion, or more specifically shifting levels of political unrest within a country or region, can have considerable impact on medical tourism flows to different destinations. For example, when there is a breakdown in a country's national governance, such as the series of political coups resulting in military rule in Thailand, the flow of medical tourists decreases. As noted in the media in 2014, "It's now 100 days since the military junta's National Council for Peace and Order (NCPO) took power in Thailand, despite numerous pleas and promotions from the Thailand Tourism Authority, the tourism industry has still not fully recovered from the effects of the government overthrow" (Cobaj 2014, n.p.).

Acts of terrorism have also become another deterrent to tourism and medical tourism alike. Many health workers discussed how the 2008 terrorism attacks in Mumbai caused the flow of international patients to decline significantly. Although few considered that the risk of terrorism was high in the nation, providers asserted that their drop in medical tourism at the time was related to the damage it inflicted on the national "brand" of India.

DISEASE OUTBREAKS: THE MOBILITY OF PATHOGENS AND PEOPLE

The emergence of a new breed of pathogenic outbreaks that have swept across the world has the potential to alter the trajectory of medical tourism, particularly for developing nations.

In addressing the topic, Singer's (2009) publication, "Pathogens Gone Wild," suggests that medical anthropology can bring new perspectives to our understandings of pandemics such as the global COVID-19 pandemic or the Swine Flu (H1N1) outbreak of 2009. Singer contends that although emergent pathogens are biological occurrences, "their appearance among humans and their health and social impacts are mediated by microsocial processes embedded within large-scale inegalitarian social structures and their environment-shaping influences" (2009, 201). Singer further posits that stigmatization related to where the pathogens first emerge, and where they are most prevalent and/or fatal, have thus far been directed toward countries in the developing world. Developing nations seeking to increase medical tourism, such as India, are rightly concerned about the damage this stigmatization brings to the international reputation of their healthcare system.

The effect of pandemics on medical tourism is evolving, with the Indian and global medical tourism industry coming to a grinding halt during the peak of the global Covid-19 pandemic. The impact of the earlier Swine Flu (H1N1 Influenza A) outbreak provides an example of the potential disruptions pandemics can cause. The first registered Swine Flu case in India was in June of 2009, in the midst of my fieldwork. Although the "pandemic" had already come and gone in many other countries with far less ferocity in terms of mortality than first envisaged, the Indian media was awash with fear-based rhetoric and imagery by early August 2009. The general picture painted was that Swine Flu was an extremely dangerous pathogen that would likely kill you if infected.

In Mumbai, after the death of two flu victims on one night shut down cinemas, colleges, and schools in the city for three to five days, with rumors circulating that the Shiv Sena had been threatening violence against any schools resisting closure. Large public celebrations, such as the Dahi Handi festivities, were also cancelled or downscaled in an attempt to reduce transmission rates. The social panic caused by the outbreak in the general population was unmistakable. The rush to buy masks led to shortages of supply across the city, with some keeping a small supply of the "high-grade" masks for themselves and their families. I saw one medical shop in Chembur selling masks for INR 500, despite their usual retail price of INR 5. There were advertisements for Ayurvedic antiswine flu treatments (including special "healing oils") advertised in every nook and cranny of the local newspapers and across popular internet sites. There were specific clinics set up to officially test for the disease, but they were regularly swamped by hordes of people waiting in long queues for hours to get tested. I continued travelling across the city during the time, spending time in Khalsa Hospital and Hospital A. During the main outbreak, I visited Khalsa to interview Colonel

Nandal. He noted that the impact of the international outbreak of Swine Flu on medical tourism in the hospital was substantial, dropping to their lowest intakes of recent years.

A short time after the Swine Flu outbreak, reports of a new, antibiotic resistant "superbug," the New Delhi Metallo-beta-lactamase-1 (NDM-1), emerged after a POI Swedish patient contracted a urinary tract infection during travel to New Delhi. Fecal samples from the patient showed the presence of an NDM-1 E. *coli*. The resistance of NDM-1 to almost all antibiotics had given cause for concern due to the risk of its potential for rapid dissemination, particularly within clinical settings. A study published in the Lancet (Kumarasamy et al. 2010) later reported on 180 cases of patients infected with NDM-1, including 37 cases in the United Kingdom and 143 cases at different sites throughout India and Pakistan. Other cases have since been reported worldwide (Rolain, Parola, and Cornaglia 2010).

When NDM-1 was first identified in India, the Indian National Centre for Disease Control denied that its outbreak was of any public health significance or concern. There were also claims in the media insinuating that it was a scare campaign designed by richer nations to dampen the medical tourism industry in India due the corresponding loss in profits in their own medical sectors (John 2011; Khandelwal 2011).

The Swine Flu outbreak was a minor precursor of the disruptive power of outbreaks of global pandemics on medical tourism. The coronavirus pandemic outbreak that developed in 2020 serves as a powerful example of how the mobility of people and pathogens can so rapidly impact on medical tourism and tourism generally. Some medical tourism centric hospitals in Malaysia and Thailand had reported drops in net profit of around 50% by mid-2020 (Kishimoto 2021). In India, hospitals in Chennai, Bengaluru, Hyderabad, and Kochi that had been heavily reliant on international patients had already recorded weighty declines in revenue by October 2020 (Rekhi and Akshatha 2020).

It is in this context that we see Appadurai's (1990) global scapes, inclusive of Inhorn's (2011) highly pertinent extension bioscapes, come to life via the global circulation and cultural flows of COVID-19. In particular, it enables a closer analysis of the pandemic's impact via its intersections across these scapes with other phenomena such as medical tourism. For example, efforts to slow the global circulation of the virus (bioscapes) significantly disrupted the ability of people to travel for medical tourism (ethnoscapes), leading to depressions in the global market and driving many of the global population into poverty (financescapes), fueled by media imagery of the global spectacle of mass infections across the world (mediascapes), and imaginaries of how medical tourism may be globally re-envisaged in post-COVID futures (ideoscapes).

CONCLUSION

The correlation between patients traveling internationally to access healthcare services to tourism is not widely acknowledged. This chapter illustrates the significance of the connections and associations of medical tourism with the broader tourism industry, tracing the functions, processes, motivations, and mechanisms used by hospitals, healthcare professionals, and government. In India, both government and providers alike understate the importance of the medical tourism sector as a vehicle to drive economic growth, yet the extent of investment is revealed in the agency of these stakeholders.

In relation to broader studies of tourism, Bianchi (2009) makes the point that it is important for critical approaches that call into question "the actions and interactions between agency and discourses, and theorization of such defensive struggles in relation to the reproduction of institutional complexes and structures of power" (Bianchi 2009, 49). This form of critical enquiry has been largely overlooked in extant studies of medical tourism. As such, this chapter has outlined the substantial associations and links of medical tourism with the broader tourism industry from the perspective of private Trust hospitals in Mumbai. These relationships are emerging in the private tertiary healthcare sector, where hospitals are transforming to attract international patients and to conform to international notions of advanced care and hospitality standards.

NOTES

1. Also known as dark or black tourism, referring to tourism in places or sites that are related to death and tragedy such as sites marking mass genocide or war.

2. Varanasi has also been known as Banaras/Benares and Kashi.

3. Shiva, alternatively known as "The Destroyer", is a Hindu god with pre-Vedic origins. A composite of multiple older gods, Shiva is viewed as the creator, protector and transformer of the universe. Married to the goddess Parvati, Shiva's children are the gods Ganesha and Kartikeya.

4. In Jainism, an ascetic monastic faith in India, Tirthankaras are believed to be the communicators of *dharma*. Both teachers and saviors, Tirthankaras are those who have 'crossed the river' of rebirth. An historical figure, Parsvanatha is the 23rd of 24 Tirthankaras, born in Varanasi in 817 BCE. Parsvanatha is thought to have first articulated the ascetic order of Jainism.

5. Bhattacharya (2013) and Arnold (1970) posit that the concept of 'tropical' was a colonial construct itself, creating imaginaries of tropical places as diseased and dangerous (Adams 2004). It was within this reframing that hill stations were cast as places of health, and urban locations as unclean, contaminating spaces.

Chapter 4

Places in Peril

Medical Tourism and the Transitioning of Trust

One of the core propositions of this book is that medical tourism contributes to local disruptions in the delivery of healthcare services to the resident population. I argue that this eventuates, in part, through its connection to the corporatization of the institutions that deliver care and the commodification of the healthcare system as a whole. There has been some scholarly focus on medical tourism and the rise of corporate tertiary healthcare conglomerates in India (Chakravarthi 2011; Lefebvre 2009, 2010). However, the role of Trust hospitals in this phenomenon has not been adequately addressed in previous research, despite the substantial number of elite Trust institutions in urban centers of India—such as Mumbai—that are engaging in the trade. Thus, this chapter focuses on the impact of medical tourism on for the Trust hospitals of Mumbai.

The period of my fieldwork (2009 to 2010) coincided with significant shifts in each of the Trust hospitals in this study, where local, national, and international market forces were driving rapid commercialization processes. Chapter 3 outlined the different marketing mechanisms employed by Trust hospitals to attract medical tourists, while highlighting their caution in acknowledging or openly professing their commercial approach. This chapter shows how the economic conditions provide a platform to encourage private institutions to operate in economic subsets that benefit the elite (Singer and Castro 2004). The chapter further outlines how Trust hospitals are shifting to this style of operation, describing the precarious economic situations of the hospitals and the significance of this to the advent of medical tourism. First, some of the difficulties of defining and tracking institutions are addressed, particularly those in the private sector. There is little compulsory public reporting required for private hospitals, which allows these institutions to avoid scrutiny of how public funds (direct and indirect) are used to secure outcomes that benefit the broader population or the national economy. Without substantial reform, the lack of transparency in the sector will encourage predatory market practices that trigger unintended consequences across the tertiary healthcare sector. This phenomenon of policy leading to unintended side effects is not specific to India; it is a well-documented occurrence globally (Allen-Scott, Hatfield, and McIntyre 2014; Koch 2014; Lehmann and Gilson 2013; Lipsitz 2012; Peters et al. 2013; Singer and Castro 2004; Smith-Oka 2009).

This chapter outlines the economic models used by Trust hospitals in the past but are no longer financially viable, even in the current context of healthcare as a booming, profitable industry. These new configurations in the charitable hospital sector are enabling "exploitative institutions to project a false image of conspicuous benevolence" (McKinlay 1985, 5) emulating similar patterns that emerged in the United States in the 1980s. Further detail is provided regarding the more significant changes taking place in the charitable hospitals in this milieu, analyzing the adaptations and transitions the hospitals of this study were in the midst of in an attempt to maintain their financial viability. Trust hospitals in India are reaching an impasse, where their former benevolent approaches are incompatible with a market-led healthcare system. As noted by Mr. Rodriguez, a senior executive at one of the Trust hospitals, "We as a Trust Hospital, we can see a stalemate coming. I've spent many years in finance, but literally, all who have given us donations are from one point in time. Today nobody will give us the same type of funds." These contradictions are intensifying, with the result that doubts are exposed about the pro-equity discourse of Trust hospitals, the wake of their shift to market led, corporate models.

In shifting to corporate modes of operation, the services offered in tertiary hospitals also change, with a greater focus on more profitable, high-end, high-tech services. Although the domestic demand for tertiary healthcare services is high in India, only a small percentage of the local population have the ability to pay for the high-end services that are emerging on the basis of this new model. This is why the sector is now looking to international patients, seeking these types of services, to fill their beds and, ultimately, maintain their ongoing financial survival.

These changes are driven by competitive practices and market expansion in the sector. The outcomes are dual-fold: growing pressure on hospitals to seek additional "consumers" outside of the domestic market, in this case, foreign medical tourists; and an expanding corporate tertiary sector that does not respond to or reflect the collective healthcare needs of the local population.

TERTIARY HEALTH CHARACTERISTICS: DISENTANGLING SECTORAL CLASSIFICATIONS

In India, hospitals are categorized via multiple classifications with regard to sector, financial governance, and function. Although the public system has defined structural classifications, the private system has far less distinct categories. The regulatory framework requires little reporting by the private sector and the absence of meaningful data means that investigation and analysis of the private sector is extremely difficult. The best available quantitative data has been generated from economic surveys of household spending in the private sector and levels of outpatient and inpatient occurrences.

In the tertiary sector of India's healthcare system, there are three main providers: public (government) hospitals, private charitable hospitals, and Corporate Hospitals. These hospitals can be further categorized as Major/General Hospitals, Super-Specialty Hospitals (e.g., cancer, heart), and Allopathic Medical Education Institutions (National Health Accounts Cell 2005; Rao et al. 2006). The first level of classification for the tertiary sector is the differentiation between hospitals located in the public and private sector. Although this delineation is clear in "theory," the increasingly complex, blended roles played by both public and private providers has created crossover in both sectors.

In the public sector, the government's involvement is increasingly complex. Although the national government owns and runs many large Major/General Hospitals, the mix between the public and private sector has become increasingly intermingled, shifting toward the use of a quasi-market model. State Health Corporations sponsored by the World Bank initiated collaborations between the public and private sector under the introduced Private Public Partnership policy. The government may own a hospital, but its management and equipment provision are contracted out to private companies. In 2001, the World Bank gave the Government of Maharashtra a USD 134 million loan, with an attached condition that 5% of this was to be used to build a corporate tertiary hospital in Mumbai. This hospital, the Wockhardt Hospital Mumbai, was built under the management of the Wockhardt Group (Yamey 2001).

The funding arrangement was a precursor to future funding in the private tertiary sector. The International Financial Corporation (IFC), the private lending branch of the World Bank Group, now regularly arranges finance for many corporate hospitals in India. In 2009, there were approximately 262 Indian healthcare services projects that had received financing from the IFC. More than 150 private corporations, including the larger healthcare, conglomerates Apollo, Max, and Fortis now have interests in hospitals across the country. Many of these are technologically driven, multi super-specialty, 100 plus bed facilities, with the vast majority located in the urban centers of the country. The dominant financial backing of these hospitals comes from financial and industrial groups (Lefebvre 2009). In September 2003, the Central Government introduced a P-P-P policy to guide future developments in the Indian healthcare sector. This policy outlined a number of measures such as: the outsourcing of management of public facilities from government to NGOs; the outsourcing of private specialist services; and the contracting out of hospital's subsidiary services (National Health Accounts Cell 2005; Rao et al. 2006). Despite initial attempts to promote affiliations between the public and private sectors, formal arrangements remain relatively *ad hoc*. The planned strategies and monitoring of the outcomes of these relationships are either weak or absent and are not publicly reported.

In the private tertiary sector, hospitals are legally differentiated by their charitable or for-profit status. This determines how the hospitals function operationally, the types of charges and/or concessions they can apply for, the rules and regulations that apply, and the out-of-pocket costs for patients. Although there are clear legal distinctions between the two, in many cases practical differentiation between charitable and corporate hospitals can be difficult to ascertain. The principal distinction between the two is that the goal of corporate hospitals is to seek profit for their shareholders, while the Trust hospitals is to seek to attain surplus to reinvest in the hospital.

There is a transformation occurring across the nation, with the growth of an industry such as medical tourism merely an indicator of such shifts. The reality for the majority of Trust hospitals in the nation in the current economic climate is to choose to either: transform their core ideals toward a market-based ethos to continue to remain viable; or allow their management to be handed over to one of the larger Healthcare conglomerates operating in the country in order to attain sufficient funding; or submit to the inevitability of being shut down. More than ever, the costs of running a hospital are rising exponentially, yet the historical means of fundraising are simply no longer sufficient. An increasing number of Trust hospitals are now transitioning. They are either moving to a market model, or they are outsourcing to corporate bodies to shift their operations and ethos to a manner similar to the corporate hospitals. For example, two of the charitable hospitals in this study already had outsourced their management to private conglomerates (charitable offshoots of major multinationals), and another was exploring new means to create additional capital through expansion of hospital bed capacity (a market-led model).

THE AMBIGUOUS CATEGORIZATION OF HOSPITALS IN MUMBAI

The five hospitals focused on for this ethnography were all situated in the private sector but are legally classified as charitable institutions. They were not selected for strategic, but rather, pragmatic reasons. When I first arrived in Mumbai for my fieldwork in early 2009, I had not yet determined the specific hospitals that would become the primary sites for this study. As I had already visited the city several months earlier on an exploratory trip to ascertain the viability of the study, I was acutely aware that this would be an ongoing process of (re)negotiation. My primary advisor and informant in India had assured me that he would be able to facilitate an entry point from which to make these negotiations. Although he had advised me that entrée would heavily depend on "who you know," I was unaware of the extent to which this would impact on the research and my ability to access key informants and accurate information.

I explained to my advisor the type of hospitals I envisioned as suitable for the study: large, private institutions that dealt with a reasonable flow of medical tourists. At the time, I was largely unaware of the significance and shifting role played by Trust hospitals across the nation. During an earlier trip to Mumbai, I had visited one such Trust hospital, which appeared to embody all of the "five-star" hotel aspects advertised by corporate hospitals. Attempting to accurately identify and understand the less obvious and more complex differences between charitable Trust hospitals, corporate hospitals, and even some of the larger public hospitals in the city, was far more fraught. Many of the hospitals' functions such as their funding, management, and operational models, often exhibit more similarities across classification lines than differences.

Through a drawn-out process of negotiation and meetings with the senior administrators, the larger number of hospitals of interest for this research was narrowed down by their willingness to participate in the research. Of course, this presents a range of limitations to the study, particularly given that none of the for-profit, corporate hospitals in the city were receptive to involvement. This has, in turn, shaped the findings of the research, revealing unexpected outcomes about the transitions taking place across the private (and public) tertiary healthcare sector in the city of Mumbai.

The hospitals studied differed significantly in their age, geographic location, reputation, management processes and ethos, and bed capacity. All five hospitals had newly updated (or updating) modern infrastructure, and two of the hospitals were built in the early years of the 2010s. The three older hospitals were all in the process of a variety of major operational and physical transformations with the intent of "turning around" the unsustainable economic positions they had found themselves in. One was in the midst of extensive renovations and extension at the time of my fieldwork, and another was in the process of constructing a multistorey tower behind the current hospital to double its bed capacity. The last of the older hospitals was in the midst of the difficult process of attempting to acquire more land to expand its bed capacity.

Two of the hospitals were registered religious Trusts and the remaining three categorized as charitable Trusts. However, the management ethos of each of the five hospitals was significantly influenced by the religions of the respective founders and Board of Trustees. The hospitals were all classified as multispecialty, ranging from 22 to 47 medical specialties. Four of the hospitals had research and development divisions, two of which were also classified as teaching institutions. They were all medium to large hospitals, with the smallest having a 230-bed capacity and the largest at 364. At the time of writing this book, the largest has managed to increase its capacity to 700 beds. The oldest hospital was first established in 1875, and the two most recent were opened in 2004 and 2005, respectively.

All five hospitals had varying engagement with medical tourism. Khalsa hospital identified its inflow of medical tourists as upward of 20% of their annual intake, but most of the other hospitals did not have specific reporting mechanisms monitoring the volume of external patients. The hospitals also attracted medical tourists from different countries or regions. This was often due to a combination of their historical, cultural, religious, or philosophical foundations. For example, Tayyib hospital predominantly attracted Dawoodi Bohra patients from Eastern bloc countries, while the more secular Ramrakhyani Hospital attracted more medical tourists from developed countries such as the United Kingdom. Sacred Heart and Ganapathiraju, both older and more established hospitals, reported that most of their medical tourists were from neighboring regions including Nepal and Bangladesh as well as northern African nations.

Dr Kakar, the Medical Director of one of the smaller and older hospitals in the study, explained that although all the corporate hospitals in the city treated high volumes of medical tourists, not all Trust hospitals were engaging with medical tourism, or at least not strategically. He explained that medical tourists coming to his hospital were primarily incidental, noting "we're not run like a business, this is like a community hospital."

Despite this, many healthcare professionals referred to different Trust hospitals in a manner that did not reflect their legal classification of

Table 4.1 Characteristics of the Hospitals (2009–10)

	Hospital A	Sacred Heart Hospital	Khalsa Hospital	Tayyib Hospital	Ramrakhyani Hospital
Trust Management	Corporate	Religious	Charitable	Religious	Charitable
Religion	Hindu	Catholic	Sikh	Dawoodi Bohra	Sindhi
Business model	Quasi-corporate	Charitable	Quasi-corporate	Quasi-corporate	Quasi-corporate
Research	✓	✓	✓	X	✓
Teaching	✓	X	✓	X	X
Nursing College	✓	X	✓	X	✓
Specialties	24	22	35	47	32
Year of establishment	1875	1942	1973	2005	2004
Bed capacity	350	232	364	259	240
Staff	258 consultants 1,000 total staff (including paramedical)	137 consultants	265 consultants. 140 resident doctors. 25 Nursing Students	700 medical staff	Unknown

Source: Fieldnotes (2021).

not-for-profit status. For example, my informants regularly referred to Khalsa, Tayyib, and Ramrakhyani hospitals as part of the corporate sector. Khalsa Hospital even has a "corporate profile" section on its website. Dr Chopra, a hospital administrator at Tayyib Hospital at one of the larger, newer hospitals, noted, "Corporate hospitals, they have this profit-making business in mind. That is their core philosophy. But in non-profit organisations here, we have safe, affordable and ethical practice of medicine." However, Dr Chopra also consistently referred to Taayib's corporate structure, management and function, and the overarching "business orientation" of the hospital's Medical Directors. Further, most people referred to the larger private hospitals catering to the elite of the city as corporate hospitals, regardless of their charitable status. However, the vast majority of the hospitals in the city, aside from public hospitals, are classified as charitable institutions, managed by Trusts.

Given that most of the larger multispecialty private hospitals in the city are classified as charitable institutions, analyzing the philosophical models espoused by each institution alongside their corporatized mode of function and governance became one of the more striking factors of this study. In an article published in 2008 in Mumbai's *Express Healthcare,* it was aptly noted, "The era of globalization and corporatization has swept trust hospitals in its wake. The end result: dingy rooms replaced by swanky interiors, unfriendly staff giving way to smiling employees and hospitals being equipped with the latest technology" (N. Singh 2008). This is particularly noteworthy in the context of the processes of hypercommodification transforming the sector.

HOSPITALS AS A SITE OF INVESTMENT

Several decades ago, McKinlay (1985) argued that the healthcare sector is highly attractive to private investors, as it is "guaranteed" to experience profit. He theorized that this was due to the vested interests of the state to ensure government underwrites its profitability, regardless of the levels of privatization. Although McKinlay was referring to the context of the United States in the 1980s, much of his analysis can be similarly applied to the healthcare setting in India in more recent years. Investment in the healthcare sector, particularly in hospitals, experienced rapid growth from the early 2000s. Investment was encouraged by the removal of all restrictive barriers for FDI in the hospital sector in 2001. This allowed foreign investors to contribute up to 100% in hospitals by an automatic route of approval. Prior to this time, there were regulatory barriers that prohibited foreign investment of

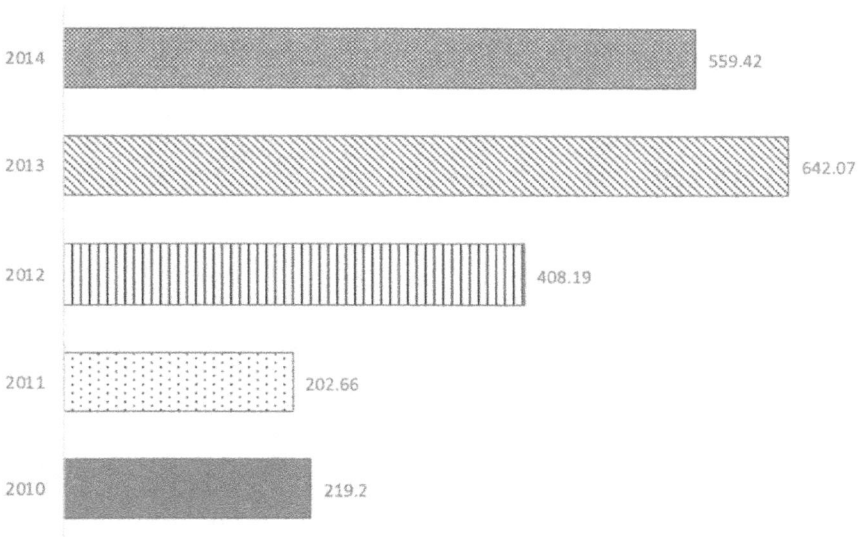

Figure 4.1   FDI in Hospitals and Diagnostic Centers (USD $ million). *Source*: Image created by author. Data from Department of Industrial Policy and Promotion (2014).

over 50%, and all FDI went through a process of government evaluation prior to approval. As illustrated by figure 4.1, between 2010 and 2014, hospital and diagnostic centers attracted approximately USD 2 billion FDI into India (Department of Industrial Policy and Promotion 2014).

In this policy context, corporate hospitals (many run by large conglomerates) have multiplied in the urban centers of the nation, typically delivering high-tech, super-specialized biomedical services provided at fees that the vast majority of the population cannot afford or access. These corporate hospitals aggressively market the new neoliberalized service industry of medical tourism, endeavoring to attract foreigners through offering health services of comparable standard and considerably lower prices to those found in the patient's country of origin. With the growth of the Indian middle class, the demand for high-end tertiary services is further driving the expansion of the sector:

Many other foreign countries and foreign investors are putting their money to the metropolitan cities in India. Because there is a class now, because of the global, this thing globalization, there is a class of people who need not, maybe they don't want to go to the government hospital because of their own reasons. Like, the care is not very good over there.

(Dr Chopra)

CHARITABLE, RELIGIOUS, AND
QUASI-CORPORATE TRUST HOSPITALS

The quality of many high-end private tertiary healthcare institutions in India are on par, if not higher, than that of most nations globally, but there is a large divide between quality and standards of care within and between the private hospitals in the country. Although a simple delineation can be made between the for-profit (corporate) and not-for-profit (Trust) hospitals, it is not necessarily accurate. As explained in chapter 3, many of the newer Trust hospitals are more closely aligned with the self-appointed "5 star" corporate hospitals in their façade, infrastructure, hospitality features, and treatment of patients. A senior consultant, Dr D'Costa, spoke openly of the different perceptions within Indian society of two prominent Trust hospitals he worked in. He noted that he treats both the elite sector and general populace using the same fee structure. However, he explained that patients such as senior politicians and Bollywood actors prefer one hospital over the other:

> I've treated the Chief Minister, VIPs, film actresses and actors, you know, they prefer to see me at Lilivati Hospital. But the common man comes and see me at the Sacred Heart, thinking that my fee structure might be different. But my fee structure for consultations is the same in the evening. But the perception - because they see these prosperities - but also as you may have gathered, the atmosphere is a lot different. There is less, what should I say; you know . . . you don't have too many uniformed staff and they conduct themselves in a manner that is like, more decorum.

Both of the hospitals referred to by Dr D'Costa were located in the same prosperous suburb of Mumbai and both have charitable trust hospital status, yet one has a reputation for much higher standards of care and higher cost. Both of the hospitals and consultants rely heavily on reputation for referral of patients. Dr Kakar, who consulted out of Sacred Heart Hospital, several other large private charitable hospitals and two corporate hospitals, explained the multitiered system, which in his opinion was far more relevant to medical tourism than the sector in which it was situated. Hospitals in the higher tiers are those that he considered to be on par with Western nations such as the United States. This included the newer charitable hospitals such as Tayyib and Ramrakhyani, but also some of the older charitable hospitals that had undergone major renovations, upgrades, and expansion of their infrastructure. He explained that there are steady flows of medical tourists seeking services in older charitable hospitals, such as Sacred Heart Hospital, but these patients were generally from developing countries seeking low-cost medical treatments inaccessible at home.

The uptake of medical tourism in these Mumbai hospitals reveals the inequities present in healthcare systems globally. The standards of what is seen as acceptable for a "foreigner" as compared to an Indian citizen is both negotiated and reinforced in these global frames of reference. This is also the case in terms of what is expected for higher and lower classes in the nation. Most private hospitals have at least three different classes of rooms, with the best rooms and care offered at the greatest expense. This can range from a cot bed in a ward room with 50 other people, through to a private room with ocean views. However, the beds sectioned off for free patients are always situated in the large wards, and often flow out into the corridors, making it difficult to even differentiate wards from overflow.

GROWTH OF THE CORPORATE
TERTIARY HEALTHCARE SECTOR

At the time of India's Independence, the private hospital sector was in its infancy, and most private hospitals were small, informal institutions, established by philanthropists. By 1974, private hospitals only represented approximately 18.5% of the tertiary health sector in India. As of 2014, it was estimated that private hospitals make up about three quarters of the tertiary sector (Hooda 2015, 2). In 2014, the business of healthcare was only about 4% of the nation's GDP, but in real terms this equated to approximately USD 81 billion. The industry has grown exponentially over recent years, increasing from USD 51 billion in 2008. Some estimates suggest the sector will grow to upward of USD 372 billion by 2022 (India Brand Equity Foundation 2021). The "market" is "booming."

With the geographic expansion of Mumbai's borders and rapid growth of suburban slums, the Brihanmumbai Municipal Corporation, who are responsible for the delivery of public tertiary healthcare services in their capacity as the local civic government, have been unable to keep up with the ever growing demand. Although some of the best public hospitals in the country are located within the city limits, there are a total of only 14 public hospitals catering to a population of over 20 million. This needs to be considered in terms of the stark reality that Mumbai is the healthcare hub for rural areas of Maharashtra and that many people travel from across the country to access the specialty services offered.

The shortfall of public hospital capacity to cater to the resident population has driven the expansion of corporate hospitals in the city's suburbs in recent decades. The Mumbai experience is also intimately linked to the rapid rise of corporate hospital networks across the nation. This has drawn criticism on multiple fronts. For example, Lefebvre (2010) described the impact of corporatization on rising patient fees.

The entry of former charitable hospitals into these networks and the medical race between hospitals to attract patients and doctors have been driving the medical cost up for the patient. The gap between corporate hospitals on one side and other private and state-run hospitals on the other side has surely increased (Lefebvre 2010, 24).

Further, increases in fees for medical services will significantly impact on the local population's access to hospitals. Hospitalization is often the most impoverishing medical service for those on or below the poverty line. This is due to the high cost of admittance, the cost of the procedure, and medicines required. Other factors incur further expenses such as the time unable to work and travel costs.

Price setting for tertiary healthcare services is driven by the private sector, which flow on to pricing in the public sector, affecting all patients. Further, fees are deregulated and lack uniformity across India. Although several national medical associations recommend costs for different services and procedures, an early study of private medical practice in India showed that only around 11% of providers follow this advice when setting their fees (Bhat 1999). This study indicated that only 47% of providers determined fees by actual costs, and a third of providers charged according to market value (Bhat 1999). The National Commission on Macroeconomics and Health (2005) also found that fees in the private sector are often "influenced by the source of capital and interest rates and prices of other inputs such as labour, rentals technology" (Ministry of Health and Family Welfare 2005, 53). Expenses in both the private and public sector have increased exponentially over past decades, where the average private cost of hospitalization has more than doubled in urban areas and has increased 42% in rural areas.

QUASI-CORPORATE HOSPITALS: THE HYPERCOMMODIFICATION OF THE NOT-FOR-PROFIT SECTOR

Philanthropy and voluntarism have long been important features of Indian civil society. Historically, this can be linked to the concept of *dharma*, which has played a central role in many Indian philosophies and religions over the course of centuries. The concepts of charity and *dharma* are also used in the interpretation of the laws of the nation (Qadeer 2000, 115). An extensive charitable sector has emerged in India over thousands of years, however, there was little organization of the sector up until the period of British colonization. The British East India Company (BEIC) founded the first, small allopathic hospital in Bombay in the late 1670s. Over a century later, the

BEIC had established only three hospitals in the city, with two being entirely dedicated for use by European troops.

It was not until the early 19th century that Christian missionaries mobilized the first organized voluntarism in social development. Primarily aimed at promoting Christianity, they built many schools, sanatoriums, dispensaries, and orphanages in urban areas. In the 1820s, a new wave of voluntarism driven by Indian elites saw the establishment of infirmaries, sanatoriums, and dispensaries in the city through philanthropic funding, some of which evolved over the years to become major hospitals (Agarwal and Dadrawala 2004).

Locally funded philanthropy was often undertaken due to coercive pressure applied by the British colonialists who were reluctant to fund health and welfare initiatives for the local population. However, this form of philanthropy was soon found to be an effective means to build the social status of local Indian donors as patrons and community leaders. The majority of these private institutions were founded with a focus on specific religious or community groups, and by the 1920s, philanthropic donors, welfare societies, and government were collaborating in the funding and management of a vast number of healthcare institutions (Kurian 2013). Many of these early Trust-run institutions were instrumental in forming the current network of the private tertiary hospitals in Mumbai today.

In the early 1800s, the growing private tertiary sector was largely unregulated. The first relevant law introduced in the area, *the Societies Act 1867*, allowed charitable bodies to register with the government. The registered charitable bodies were then later enabled access to tax incentives after the introduction of the *Income Tax Act* in 1921 (S. Sen 1992). In Maharashtra, the *Bombay Public Trusts Act (BPT)* was introduced in 1950, setting out the legal requirements for registered Trusts in the state. Under this legislation, Trusts may register as either public or private organizations and are further categorized as religious or charitable.

Under section 41AA of the BPT, Trusts that run charitable or religious hospitals are legally required to set aside 10% of their total hospital beds for the "indigent" sector free of any charge for health services. They are also required to provide a further 10% of their beds for the economically weaker sector (EWS) at a subsidized cost. Under the Act, the "indigent" sector (SC/ST) is classified as those earning less than INR 50,000 (USD 750) annually. The EWS is defined as those earning an annual income in the range of INR 50,000 to one lakh[1] (USD 1,500). It is the requirement of charitable hospitals to establish an Indigent Patient's Fund (IPF). The BPT Act stipulates that this fund must only be used to cover the costs related to treatment of the indigent and weaker sector. The hospital's Trust must credit the fund with 2% of the billing of all patients on a monthly basis. Any donations to the hospital must also be applied to the IPF.

In 2013, the Charity Commissioner of Maharashtra reported a total of 80 registered charitable hospitals in Mumbai, with a combined total of 7,580 beds. Across all 80 hospitals, 751 beds are required to be reserved for the indigent sector and another 781 to the EWS (Charity Commissioner of Maharashtra n.d.). Of the 80 charitable hospitals, the vast majority are smaller institutions, with the 25 largest hospitals accounting for approximately 85% of the beds (Charity Commissioner of Maharashtra n.d.). In 2013, 14 charitable hospitals made an appeal to the Charity Commissioner to suspend the treatment of free patients citing financial difficulties (Kurian 2013, 3). Khalsa, Tayyib, and Ramrakhyani Hospitals were among the 14 appellants. As an outcome of the appeal, the Charity Commissioner issued a directive allowing four of the hospitals to cease providing free treatments temporarily, including Khalsa Hospital and Ramrakhyani Hospital. In a discussion with Dr Lulla in 2009, he insisted that Ramrakhyani Hospital was not under any obligation to provide free treatment for poorer patients, but they did so because of the hospital's "ethos":

> We know that a lot of people can't afford us. So, we have a charity department, so people who can't afford, we set aside 2% of our gross earnings. To help them, we have done heart valve replacements and transplants, everything for free. That focus is more of an individual ethos. I don't know how many people would do it because they would have to ensure sustainability of their organization. So, we ensure that we do have such people also.

Several hospitals in the study had been under investigation for failure to comply with the BPT Act. In Duggal's (2012) article "The Uncharitable Trust Hospitals," he argued that Trust hospitals consistently breach the BPT Act and that many of the hospitals use the BPT Act merely to access the tax incentives and other related benefits, failing to comply with the required quota of "free" patients. Duggal estimated the annual gross profit made by the Trust hospitals in Mumbai to be over USD 150 million, yet the cost of providing free and low-cost beds for the poor amounts to under USD 34 million. This shortfall of USD 116 million should be viewed as a direct government subsidy to the private Trust hospitals.

Drawing on data sourced from the Maharashtra Charity Commissioner's Office, Kurian's (2013) review of Trusts Hospitals of Mumbai assessed their compliance with the BPT Act. The findings were damning, as most charitable hospitals were noncompliant with the Act. Key areas of concern included the failure of 98% of hospitals to allocate the required percentage of beds for the disadvantaged and the misreporting and underreporting of philanthropic donations and bed numbers. Further, the report noted that the Indigent Patients Fund (IPF) is underutilized in all hospitals despite complaints from the major Trust hospitals that they cannot afford to implement the scheme. Last, the study noted the insufficient monitoring of compliance with the Act. Even when hospitals were found to be in breach of the Act, no disciplinary action has been initiated. Similar breaches of regulatory requirements by private hospitals have transpired across the nation. For example, the Delhi High Court panel found in 2009 that the Apollo Hospital in New Delhi was not fulfilling its regulatory requirement of providing at least a third of its beds to the disadvantaged.

HISTORICAL CONTEXT OF TRUST HOSPITALS IN MUMBAI

Given the rising economic and regulatory burdens faced by charitable institutions, the continued presence of Trust hospitals as the most prevalent providers of Mumbai's private tertiary sector can be understood through the lens of a specific set of contextual historical conditions. Fueled by internal migration, Mumbai's population expanded rapidly after India's Independence. The rapid population growth led to high population densities in the southern areas of the city, which resulted in the expansion and development of the northern areas of the city. Residential and capital flows to the northern suburbs intensified in the 1970s and 1980s; and by 1991, only 30% of the population was located in the southern area of the city (Madhiwalla 2003).

Up until the mid to late 1980s, the majority of the private healthcare sector in Mumbai consisted of single practitioners, and secondary hospitals operated and managed by charitable and religious trusts. When the New Economic Policy (NEP) was introduced in the early 1990s, the Indian government instituted expansive economic incentives to encourage greater private investment in the tertiary healthcare sector. Incentives included direct and indirect tax reductions and waivers, such as higher rates of depreciation and import duty exemptions for medical equipment, municipal and income tax exemptions, and subsidized, preferential land allocations for hospitals. Charitable hospitals also received additional subsidized costs for utilities such as electricity and water.

The lack of physical space in central Mumbai and shortage of hospitals to service the growing population facilitated the expansion of corporate hospitals in the city's northern suburbs, particularly over the past decade. As larger for-profit institutions began to infiltrate the city, smaller institutions found it increasingly difficult to compete (Sengupta and Nundy 2005).

The majority of hospitals in Mumbai's private sector are registered as charitable or religious Trusts, but many are operating under great financial strain. Others have completely altered their governance and organizational structures to a quasi-corporate framework, particularly those emerging as extremely exclusive institutions backed by the corporate sector by various mechanisms. The hospitals attracting the majority of medical tourists in the city were the corporate and the charitable, quasi-corporate hospitals, seeking to increase their profitability. The hospitals focused on for this study were all legally deemed charitable hospitals under the BPT Act, with four of the five functioning within a quasi-corporate framework. Sacred Heart Hospital was the only hospital that had not yet transitioned to this emerging economic model.

The Sacred Heart Hospital was initially established as a small 10-bed nursing home in 1942. In 1953, the nursing home expanded to 22 beds and was taken over by the Medical Mission Sisters. In 1978, the management of the nursing home was taken over by the Order of Ursuline Sisters of Mary Immaculate. The Order originated in Italy and first came to India in the early 1930s at a time when many Christian missionaries were establishing themselves across the nation, building healthcare facilities, orphanages, and schools. Over the years, the hospital has expanded to a 232-bed institution, located on the coast in West Mumbai. From an extremely humble beginning, the hospital now finds itself nestled amongst the city's elite.

Of the five hospitals, Sacred Heart had the lowest flow of international patients but had an annual inpatient turnover of between 12 and 16 thousand people. It was also the only hospital of the three older institutions that did not have extensive renovations underway. The hospital was experiencing high levels of economic strain due to the changing structure of the healthcare market in Mumbai and was undergoing significant strategic planning in an attempt to increase its competitiveness while maintaining its socio-religious ethos.

Mr. Rodriguez, the Chief Financial Officer (CFO) of Sacred Heart Hospital explained that the rise of corporate hospitals in the city was driven by corporate entities taking over the management of economically struggling Trust hospitals. One such example is the case of Raheja Hospital, a 280-bed charitable facility located in South Mumbai. Raheja hospital provided many advanced specialty services and was well-known as one of the most affordable hospitals in the city. In 2009, it was speculated that Raheja was on the brink of closure due to financial insolvency and labor issues, when it was taken over by Fortis Healthcare. Fortis Healthcare is one of the largest corporate healthcare organizations in India, with 36 healthcare facilities and over 400 diagnostic services located across the larger cities of the nation.

Mr. Rodriguez explained that although the older, established Trust hospitals in the city were struggling to maintain viability, the potential profits that could be derived from medical tourism was no panacea for most in the sector. A major barrier to accessing this market was that charitable hospitals rarely offered the specialized advanced care often sought by medical tourists, in comparison to the services offered by dedicated corporate centers such as the Asian Heart Institute.

Another factor raised by several hospital executives in the context of their financial viability was the unsustainability of the escalating tariffs for essential utilities required to run the hospitals. For example, electricity is a major operational cost faced by all Mumbai hospitals. The local municipal government body manages electricity in the state and all hospitals in the ward pay the same rate, regardless of status (public, charitable, or corporate). The tariffs paid by hospitals are marginally lower than industrial and other commercial businesses but significantly higher than residential rates. Numerous charitable trust hospitals in the city have instituted electricity saving measures, such as only air-conditioning specific areas of the hospital in an attempt to keep down costs. Incremental increases to the price of electricity instituted by BMC have had a significant impact on the viability of charitable hospitals such as Sacred Heart Hospital, in some instances more than doubling in the span of a month.

THE QUASI-CORPORATE TRANSITIONING OF GANAPATHIRAJU HOSPITAL

As outlined in the Introduction of the book, Ganapathiraju Hospital was first established during British colonial rule and the early days of the city's economic expansion. A successful Indian businessman and philanthropist who had already been involved in the establishment of a Sanatorium and a girls' school, bequeathed the extensive property from his estate to be set aside to establish a hospital in his name for the people of the city. The original hospital had a 40-bed capacity, with half of the beds allocated as non-fee paying for those unable to afford hospital fees. As demand for the hospital's services grew over the course of the 20th century, so too did the hospital, expanding to what is now a 350-bed capacity.

During the course of the 1990s, Ganapathiraju Hospital found itself in considerable financial debt. The hospital's management, not wanting to reduce the number of free beds for those unable to pay, made the decision to add additional paid beds to the hospital to increase its revenue, and in turn increase their ability to cross-subsidize care for patients. Plans were initiated to build a 19-storey building on the land directly behind the hospital. The plans were drawn up, and the building was well under way when it became apparent that the Hospital Trust did not have the funds to complete the building. The partially built multistorey tower sat unfinished behind the existing hospital for over a decade. In December 1997, the philanthropic arm of a large Indian owned multinational conglomerate signed a Memorandum of Understanding (MoU) with the Trustees of Ganapathiraju Hospital. One of the principal elements of the MoU was the agreement to transfer the Hospital's central management to the corporation's philanthropic organization, with the managing director of the corporation joining the Hospital's Board of Directors. This agreement was made due to the corporation's promise of significant capital outlay to resume building the unfinished hospital extension. Dr Nayar explained, "it's because we got stuck, we didn't have the money. So that is when [the corporation]…they came to the help of the hospital."

Initially a textile business in the 1950s, the multinational corporation has grown to engage in a range of industries including oil, gas, energy, financial services, insurance, telecommunications, and information technology. In 2021, the head of the company was listed as the wealthiest person in Asia and the 6th wealthiest person in the world. As of March 2021, he had reportedly amassed a personal fortune of approximately USD 84.5 billion (Karmali 2021). Despite this success, there have been allegations of corrupt and manipulative practices, with the corporation using its connections with bureaucrats and politicians to influence "government rules, manipulating the stock markets, and taking advantage of loopholes in the laws such as the complicated Indian taxation laws." (Kazmi 2008, 1158).

In 2001, five years after signing the MoU with Ganapathiraju Hospital, the conglomerate launched its first corporate health branch of the group, focusing on biopharmaceuticals, clinical research, regenerative medicine, molecular medicine, biofuels, plant and industry biotechnology, and pharmaceuticals. The initial intention of the establishment of the corporate health branch was to undertake research on biopolymers for the corporation. However, as the health branch grew, the two largest sources of profit, human plasma products and pharmaceuticals, became its primary focus. In 2002, the corporate health branch set up their base and a laboratory in Ganapathiraju Hospital, conducting clinical research and establishing a stem cell repository. By 2005, the health company had expanded, moving their base out of the hospital to a facility in Navi Mumbai. Indian business analysts have contended that the health group emerged as one of the highest value subsidiary companies in the Indian multinational conglomerate (Layak and Shukla 2012).

Comparable corporate diversification processes emerged in the United States healthcare sector in the mid-1970s. Salmon (1984) noted that during this period, many hospitals were restructured using corporate models and diversified their business operations, adding "new lines of business," including

Hospice care for the terminally ill, occupational medicine programs, sports medicine clinics, biomedical engineering businesses, mobile diagnostic units, alcoholic recovery centers, clinical labs, surgi-centers, dialysis centers, nursing homes, home health care, housing for the elderly, restaurants, parking lots, health spas, flower shops, shopping centers, and more. (Salmon 1984, 156–57)

Salmon contended that this diversification was a major factor that led to the blurring of lines between the charitable and corporate sectors of tertiary healthcare in the United States, of which the experience of Ganapathiraju Hospital's partnership with their corporate-philanthropic partner closely aligns.

As of early 2010, Ganapathiraju Hospital's corporate–philanthropic partner had invested over USD 15 million in the hospital, primarily for the expansion and renovation of the buildings. Shortly after my fieldwork, the hospital closed its doors for approximately 12 months to complete the major construction works. In 2014, the new hospital building was inaugurated at a grandiose ceremony, attended by Prime Minister Narendra Modi and a long list of Indian celebrities. The hospital has since promoted its "cutting-edge," "global" technologies including the use of Google Glass to track patient histories during surgery. The health subsidary of the multinational conglomerate also continued to prosper, expanding the sales of its pharmaceuticals to the United States after receiving approval from the US Food and Drug Administration (FDA) (Dandekar 2016).

The quasi-corporate transitioning of Ganapathiraju Hospital provides an important example highlighting the ever more frequent partnering of large corporations with charitable hospitals. Although the corporate–philanthropic partnership ensured that Ganapathiraju Hospital maintained its functioning—and subsequent expansion and "globalization" of its operations—the economic dividends for the multinational group has gained very little critical attention. The multinational's philanthropic engagement with Ganapathiraju Hospital provided the opportunity for corporate reputation-washing, alongside the highly profitable expansion of its business portfolio by leveraging the hospital to establish and build its health subsidary. From this perspective, the role and intent of the corporate–philanthropic partner could be viewed as less an act of beneficence, and more one of wielding power and building profitability. Hay and Muller (2014) label such forms of philanthropic activity (philanthropy of the "super" rich) as super or elite philanthropy. They suggest that different forms of super-philanthropy can also be viewed as "diverting attention and resources away from the failings of contemporary manifestations of capitalism" (Hay and Muller 2014, 648–49), whilst also transferring responsibility for public services (such as healthcare) away from government to the rich, which are then directed by the elite. These processes reinforce the local hypercommodification of the tertiary healthcare sector, which in turn, perpetuates further inequity within and across the healthcare system.

LOCAL CONTEXTUAL FORCES AND THE HYPERCOMMODIFICATION OF TRUST HOSPITALS

Another case-study highlighting the emergence of an elite, quasi-corporate Trust hospital, is that of Tayyib Hospital. Its establishment and longer history reveal a highly contested, but very different process to that experienced at Ganapathiraju Hospital. Tayyib Hospital is positioned in one of the most sought-after locations in Mumbai, overlooking one of the most popular beach promenades at the southern end of the city. The area's popularity means that it is extremely congested, even by Mumbai standards. The 14-storey palatial building juts out conspicuously above the coastal skyline, appearing somewhat removed from the clamor of the city below. It is a striking building, with a pastel peach and white exterior, portals, domes, arches, and windows influenced by the Fatimid era of architecture. The hospital has a staff of approximately 700 medical professionals and a total of 259 beds, assigning approximately 30% to disadvantaged groups within the population. An Islamic Shia subsect, the Dawoodi Bohras, built the USD 35 million hospital in 2005. Although only constructed in recent times, there is a long and contentious history relating to the ownership and management of the land and property dating back to 1886 that are intimately tied to the hospital's contemporary operations. The controversies derive from altercations between the fundamentalist and reformist groups within the Dawoodi Bohras.

Given the Hospital's prime location, I had initially speculated on how it was that such a large area of land had been made available to build a Trust hospital. During discussions with a multiple informants, with and without connections to the hospital, it became apparent there had been ongoing disquiet regarding the building, the ownership and the functioning of the religious Trust bodies related to the hospital. The concerns were primarily related to issues within the religious community that own and operate the hospital, the land it has been developed on, and the entwined socio-religious reformism that had emerged over decades.

In 1886, the land on which the current hospital stands was leased to a wealthy local philanthropist for 99 years. On the leased land, he built a *masjid* and a large Sanatorium consisting of three wings. The philanthropist, although originating from a modest, uneducated background in Gujarat, migrated to Bombay and earned the majority of his great wealth as a cotton manufacturer, selling tents and military uniforms to the British Army at the time of the Second Boer War (Roychowdhury 2009). The local philanthropist was a member of Mumbai's Dawoodi Bohras community, a minority Shi'a Muslim sect known for being progressive, educated, and business oriented.

The global Dawoodi Bohra's population is approximately one million, with the vast majority of the group living in India and Pakistan. From 1840 onward, the Dawoodi Bohras have experienced schisms, with a reformist movement shifting away from the orthodox majority. One of the key issues of consternation for the reformists is related to the complex nature of the Dawoodi Bohra doctrines. Disputes have also arisen regarding the successions of their religious leader, known as the Da'i-el-Mutlaq or Syedna (Wright Jr 1975). The Syedna holds considerable direct power and control over the community, including the right to excommunicate community members. In the past, this has primarily been used to excommunicate individuals leading reformist movements.

Notably, the descendants of the Hospital's philanthropic founder are aligned with the most recent reformist movement that followed a dispute soon after his death in 1913. A disagreement between the newly appointed Syedna and the philanthropist's sons initially arose over who should be the principal representative of the community in negotiations with the British Raj. Over time, this dispute eventuated in a range of court actions. During this period, the Syedna began a process of consolidating his economic resources using a variety of tactics, such as the collection of religious tithes, and by persuading wealthy members of the Dawoodi congregation to confer the deeds of their Trusts to him. These actions drew further criticism from the reformist movement, indignant about the unaccountability and lack of transparency in his financial dealings. One well-known academic reformist has accused the Syedna of creating "a personal religious empire" through his amassed fortune accumulated via totalitarian control (Wright Jr. 1975, 24).

In 1927, the Bombay High Court sanctioned the land and buildings of the hospital as a charitable Trust, named after the philanthropist. The Trustees were primarily the descendants of the original philanthropist, and were also reformist Dawoodi Bohras. Only three years after the Trust was established, it was declared bankrupt but was bailed out by the Tayyib Hospital Society. The Tayyib Hospital Society primarily consisted of the Syedna's family and close friends, who were then installed as the hospital Trustees. In 1944, one of the wings of the Sanatorium was temporarily chartered to the Polish Red Cross to establish a war hospital. At the behest of the Syedna, the hospital continued to operate after the departure of the Red Cross, under the sanction of the Tayyib Hospital Society. At this time hospital services were exclusively provided to the Dawoodi Bohra community, although this mission later expanded to a principle of providing "care for all." In 1973, the Tayyib Hospital Society was officially registered as a Trust, operating alongside the original hospital Trust (Engineer 1979, 964).

In 1965, the Tayyib Hospital Trust filed a petition to the Bombay Municipal Corporation Civil Court requesting permission to demolish the buildings on the property. They intended to build a new hospital in its place that would broaden the access to its services to the entire population. At the time, the 4,826 square foot property was still legally owned by the original hospital Trust, with an estimated worth of US $45 million. The property included the Tayyib Hospital, a sanatorium, a mosque, two rundown buildings, and the tomb of the original philanthropist. The petition was met with opposition from the great-grandsons of the philanthropist, who argued that the demolition would be a desecration of the tomb of their descendent. They further contended that the Tayyib Hospital Trust had engaged in deed tampering and other financial misrepresentation, matters of which remain unresolved.

After many years of litigation, the Supreme Court of India reached the finding that the Tayyib Hospital Trust was to be allowed to demolish the majority of the buildings. However, this was under the provision that another Sanatorium was built as a wing of the new hospital, inclusive of the tomb of the philanthropist. The court also ordered that 30 of the hospital's beds were to be reserved, free of charge, for members of the Dawoodi Bohra community. The Sanatorium was demolished in 2000, and construction for the new Tayyib Hospital began. Significant splits remained in the Dawoodi Bohra community regarding the signage and naming of the hospital and attached Sanatorium. There are also ongoing internal reservations in the community concerning the revenue raising for the hospital by the Syedna.

Tayyib Hospital functions within a corporate governance model, outsourcing its auditing, taxation, and advisory services to KPMG India. As a standard, there were approximately 30 foreigners (including NRIs) treated at the hospital at any given time, with four to five new patients admitted daily as a minimum during the time of fieldwork. The majority of medical tourists originated from Africa, the Middle East, Tanzania, Kenya, South Africa, the United Kingdom, the United States, Dubai, and Oman. The Administrative Manager, Ms. Chatterjee explained that the hospital has affiliations with the Oman Consulate and the Japanese Consulate to bring additional medical tourists to the hospital. One of their specialties at the hospital is in advanced robotic surgery, which attracts many foreign patients from neighboring regions that do not have access to the same biotechnology in their home countries. It is also the top hospital in the state for cadaver organ donations for transplant.

As outlined in this short history of Tayyib Hospital, although the institution has emerged as a new quasi-corporate hospital in recent years, the impetus for this transformation was not an issue of financial mismanagement forcing the transition, as that experienced by Ganapathiraju Hospital. Instead, Tayyib hospital took on a corporate management structure as a consequence of local issues of power that unfolded between members of the particular religious subsect. The power of the Syedna in his capacity to maintain and extend the hospital's philanthropic financing through specific religious practices also placed the hospital in a better position than that of other Trust hospitals in the city. This does not entirely remove its quasi-corporate transition from the frame of the hypercommodification of the wider sector, but highlights the moderated significance in this instance.

IMPACTS OF THE CORPORATIZATION
OF THE TERTIARY HEALTH SECTOR

Trends of corporatization in the tertiary health sector have been experienced in many varied countries across the world over the past five decades, including the United States, the United Kingdom, Germany, and Malaysia. The experiences of these nations could be used to inform and guide Indian policy makers to potentially avoid some of the more significant and hazardous consequences for the Indian healthcare system. By example, in the United States similar trends of corporatization occurred throughout the 1970s, with the formation of powerful corporate hospital lobby groups that successfully influenced both the regulatory and policy framework of the nation. These groups weakened areas such as reimbursement levels for the national social insurance scheme and the social healthcare program, building sanctions for hospitals, and redirected the flow of research funding to focus on corporate healthcare (Chakravarthi 2011).

Barraclough (1997) also described a similar process in Malaysia, where many of the charitable hospitals and other small private hospitals originally set up by medical professionals were absorbed by corporate conglomerates in the mid-1990s. In this context, corporatization also caused significant pressure on charitable hospitals. Many found they were unable to compete with corporate hospitals when using the cross-subsidization model that formerly enabled them to provide services for the poor (Barraclough 1997, 657).

In a review of previous decades of changes to the United States healthcare system, Himmelstein and Woolhandler (2008) have described some of the most problematic, unintended outcomes of the highly corporatized system:

> The U.S. experience also demonstrates that market mechanisms nurture unscrupulous medical businesses and undermine medical institutions unable or unwilling to tailor care to profitability. The commercialization of care in the United States has driven up costs by diverting money to profits and by fueling a vast increase in management and financial bureaucracy, which now consumes 31 percent of total health spending (Himmelstein and Woolhandler 2008, 408).

There is an underlying assumption within Indian healthcare policy that continuing the marketization of the system will provide a solution for the provision of care to the vulnerable sectors of the population. The 2010 United Nations' Mumbai Human Development Report argued that further P-P-P ventures will improve healthcare services for the poor:

> Charitable institutions have always played a seminal role in providing afford-able healthcare in Mumbai. Now there is a greater need to tap the potential for public-private partnership and community-provider linkages to strengthen the delivery mechanism of health services in Mumbai (United Nations Development Program 2010, foreword)

Instead, I contend that the experiences of the United States healthcare commodification process should be heeded as a strong warning against facilitating the control of the sector by the private market, particularly in the absence of strong, enforceable regulations, backed by political will to protect the population from further disastrous effects beyond that already experienced.

CONCLUSION

This chapter described how in past decades, many of the older Trust hospitals have acted as institutions of resilience and opposition to global structural forces that have driven the hypercommodification of the healthcare system in India. However, it is unlikely these hospitals will continue to survive without significant adaptation to make them more competitive in the corporatizing market. Many are already transitioning by modernizing and expanding their physical infrastructure, increasing their specialties and introducing advanced medical technologies. Others are changing their governance structures by partnering with corporate groups to manage their institutions in the hope that this will bring the capital and expertise required to maintain their competitiveness in the tertiary healthcare market. Although these changes may serve to secure their financial viability, they are heralding paradigmatic shifts for the charitable sector. The local interpretations, manifestations, and transformations underway in the sector in Mumbai are indicative of broader shifts within the healthcare system in India. Mr. Rodriguez emphasized the fraught circumstance for Trust hospitals in Mumbai, "Hospitals have to go ahead, otherwise, if you stand where you are, you'll be taken over by somebody else." Mr. Rodriguez, like many other hospital administrators, was pragmatic about the economic conundrum forced upon the philanthropic and religious hospitals of the city.

Through the description of the transitional processes experienced by two of the hospitals in the study, one through its partnership with a major industry conglomerate and the other through the power contests between internal factions of the religious Trust, this chapter has illustrated how market forces can influence the development and operations of different individual hospitals. However, in the different contextual settings of each hospital, it is clear that the changes to infrastructure, introduction of new biotechnologies, and shifts in governance models have made them far more competitive in the local and international market. These transitions have ensured that the individual hospitals used as case study examples are consequently less vulnerable to the market forces that plague many other charitable hospitals of the city.

As the sector continues to corporatize, shifting governance models away from a "Robin Hood" cross-subsidization model, many of the hospitals that have served the disadvantaged population are less willing to open their doors for all. This is compounded by a lack of will by government bodies, such as the Charity Commissioner, to enforce the regulatory obligations of hospitals. These factors are indicative of far more problematic issues of corruption across the nation, such as described in fine detail by Gupta (2012) in his book, *Red Tape: Bureaucracy, Structural Violence and Poverty in India*. Gupta (2012) situated the poverty experienced in India within a frame of structural violence, which is inflicted on the poor by "not only the elites but also the fast-growing middle-class, whose increasing number and greater consumer power are being celebrated by an aggressive global capitalism" (Gupta 2012, 22). Gupta further theorized that the unintentional bureaucratic modes by which this structural violence is exercised is a form of "thanatopolitics," which he argues should be understood as "killing rather than simply as allowing to die or exposing to death." (2012, 17).

Expanding on Gupta's re-envisaging of structural violence, I argue that the state's neglect of public healthcare and the concurrent hypercommodification of Trust hospitals, should be understood as another form of thanatopolitical structural violence against the poor of the nation. When Trust hospitals are reconfigured as sites that prioritize healthcare for the wealthy local population and international patients, and the state fails to provide alternative accessible services, the poor are progressively and systematically alienated from access to hospital services entirely. The structural violence inflicted on the poor has never been more evident than during the first two years of the Covid-19 pandemic. Viruses do not differentiate along socio-economic lines, yet access to potentially lifesaving healthcare in India most certainly does.

NOTE

1. Term used in Indian Numerical System. One crore is equal to one hundred thousand.

Chapter 5

Mobility, Identity, and the Global Imaginary

The Worlding of the Healthcare Workforce

Following on from the focus on the hospitals hosting medical tourism in Chapter Four, this chapter recasts our gaze to the impact of medical tourism on the health workers of Mumbai. It does so by describing and analyzing the engagement of the local Indian healthcare workforce with discourses of neoliberal development and the transformational, territorial logics of power that are reinforced by an emphasis on medical tourism. The growth of primarily medically trained Indian medical entrepreneurs has driven much of the growth of medical tourism across the nation. Many doctors in India supplement their years of medical training with master's degrees in hospital administration or general business administration to enable career progression and, in some cases, to simply maintain employment in the healthcare system. In this context, the perspectives of healthcare providers are distorted, with medicine reconfigured to a predominantly commercial venture that is unattainable for the majority of the Indian population.

The chapter demonstrates how health professional's imaginaries of the expectations of a "global patient" are translated and embedded into professional practice, drawing on Appadurai's conception of ideoscapes. Medical tourism has contributed to optimistic social and medical imaginaries of many healthcare workers, with doctors and administrators envisioning themselves as active agents via their professional contributions to shifting global perceptions of India.

The processes of healthcare hypercommodification, hospital corporatization, and increased transnational mobility have significantly impacted the lives and professional roles of the local medical workforce in Mumbai. With the shortage of medical personnel in India, education and credentialing characteristics of the medical workforce of India have emerged as key issues affecting the quality of service and the standing and morale of the workforce.

These factors are in turn influenced by the Indian diaspora, the value placed on the significance of overseas education, and the implications of different forms of mobility on healthcare workers, the interchanges and flows of people, power, and knowledge systems.

The economic drivers of the diverse forms of development and territorial logics of power deeply impact on the everyday roles of healthcare professionals. One of the features emerging from the rapid and extreme hypercommodification of the Indian healthcare system has been the shifting status and hierarchy of doctors, nurses, and hospital administrators in the context of a market-led model. An important feature of note is the relative rise of the hospital administrator within the social power dynamics of the healthcare system.

Navarro (1988) outlined similar changes to the medical workforce in the United States in the late 1980s, arguing, "physicians increasingly feel that their autonomy is being forcefully challenged by nondoctors" (Navarro 1988, 59). Although not the experience for all my informants, many within the younger generations of doctors who were less established in their fields were particularly vulnerable to these new forms of power relations. Their aspirations and deep anxieties were entangled within these rapidly transforming structures of power relations within the Indian tertiary healthcare system, leaving them to manage the precarious balance between their upward mobility and increasing precarity in the system. As a consequence, the younger generations are progressively pushed toward acquiring business and hospital administration qualifications to manage this precarity.

In this milieu, medical tourism has also presented itself as a vehicle of hope for some doctors, representing a stage from which they can showcase their "world-class" expertise and talent to a global audience. In doing so, internalized perceptions of the failure of being "left behind" by other colleagues who have migrated to "greener" Western pastures are challenged. These doctors remained intensely aware of the limitations of the local embeddedness of this "stage," with hospital infrastructural improvements, the international standardization of the national workforce and reconfigurations of sectoral power logics looming large.

In part, this chapter outlines the historical trajectory and current place and role of the medical professional in the tertiary sector in India within broader cultural and socioeconomic hierarchies, including the importance of economic factors to maintaining their status. Yet it also draws attention to implications of the paradigmatic shift away from a philanthropic medical professionalism toward a market-based ethos for the medical workforce. I conclude the chapter with two case studies that highlight specific features of the intensively hierarchical and competitive structure of the hospitals. Examples of day-to-day interactions in the hospitals reveal the importance of the medical patronage system, governance styles, and the global medical imaginaries that have emerged as central drivers for healthcare professionals in the industry.

THE INDIAN MEDICAL WORKFORCE: DEVELOPMENT OF PROFESSIONAL STANDARDS

In a study of the Indian medical workforce, Karan and others (2019) estimated that there were 0.94 million registered biomedical doctors and 1.67 million registered nursing and midwifery personnel across India in 2015 (Karan et al. 2019). The WHO (2020b) has reported the density of the Indian workforce at 0.69 physicians and 1.73 nurses and midwifery personnel per 1,000 people (see figure 5.1). These density ratios fall far short of international minimum density recommendations and are significantly lower than most nations engaging in medical tourism (see figure 5.1). The WHO has recommended that an additional 1.8 million doctors, nurses, and midwives

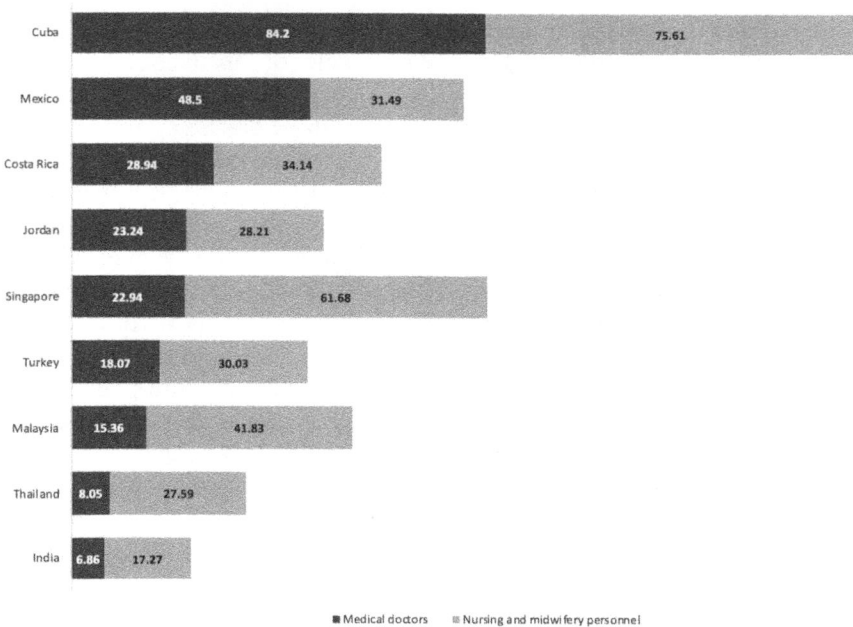

	Medical doctors	Nursing and midwifery personnel
Cuba	84.2	75.61
Mexico	48.5	31.49
Costa Rica	28.94	34.14
Jordan	23.24	28.21
Singapore	22.94	61.68
Turkey	18.07	30.03
Malaysia	15.36	41.83
Thailand	8.05	27.59
India	6.86	17.27

Figure 5.1   Healthcare Workforce Density in Medical Tourism Destinations 2018* (Per 10,000 People) *Data is reported for 2018, with the exception of Jordan, Singapore, and Malaysia. For these nations, the latest data reported for Jordan, 2017; Singapore, 2016; Malaysia, 2015. *Source*: Image created by author. Data from the WHO (2020).

are needed to achieve the minimum threshold needed in the nation (WHO 2020c).

Further, these data are only a rough estimate of the actual healthcare workforce, given calculations are based on reported registrations of healthcare workers. The genuine situation is far graver, as many registered workers no longer actively participate in the workforce. Past Indian Government reports have indicated that up to 70% of registered doctors are no longer active and many unregistered healthcare workers continue to work in the sector (Panda 2013).

Although these pronounced shortages are of great concern, the ratios have gradually improved over time. In the decade leading to India's Independence, there were only 0.16 trained doctors per 1,000 population (Rao et al. 2011). At this time, there were very few medical education institutions and no regulatory mechanisms controlling qualifications in the sector. The two qualifications available for doctors were a five and a half year medical degree for registered biomedical physicians, or a three to four year course for licentiate medical practitioners. The majority of trained doctors fell into the latter category. Shortly after India's Independence, the government of the time abolished the licentiate course, barring doctors holding this qualification from continuing in licensed practice (Rao et al. 2011). To be registered as a medical physician, doctors need to hold a Bachelor of Medicine and Bachelor of Surgery (MBBS) degree. However, given the nation's acute deficiency of trained professionals, many doctors have continued practicing with little or no formal medical training.

In a 2005 study commissioned by the World Bank on medical practice in New Delhi, Das Gupta and Rani (2004, 6) found that only around half of the visits to practitioners were with those that held an MBBS degree. Another study by Rao, Bhatnagar, Berman, Saran, and Raha (2009) concluded that untrained doctors make up to one quarter of the entire workforce, with even higher rates in rural areas. In studies focusing on rural healthcare provision, the results indicate that the numbers of unqualified healthcare practitioners are even higher. A household survey conducted in rural regions found that over 70% of visits to healthcare providers were made to unqualified practitioners and that these practitioners outweigh qualified providers 15 to 1 (Das et al. 2012). Beyond the rural–urban divide, the maldistribution of unqualified practitioners between different states and territories is significant. For example, nearly three quarters of doctors in the private sector in Assam have no registered qualifications, but in the states of Maharashtra and Gujarat, over 90% of doctors hold an MBBS (Das and Hammer 2005).

A similar development trajectory was experienced in the profession of nursing. Over time, the government has worked toward standardizing nursing education with an aim to raise the national standards of professional and clinical practice, which is highly variable across the nation. During the British occupation, medical missionaries were the first to attempt to professionalize the role, setting up many nursing schools in the southern states to train poor local women. The three main qualifications for nurses now offered in India are a three-and-a-half-year diploma in general nursing and midwifery, a four-year bachelor's degree in nursing, and a two-to-three-year postgraduate degree in nursing (Rao et al. 2011).

The majority of nursing courses are provided by private institutions, with almost 90% of all institutions situated in the private sector (Walton-Roberts 2015, 375). However, the quality of training provided by these institutions was questioned by a study commissioned by the Ministry of Health and Family Welfare that found that the majority (61.2%) failed to meet the advised standards set by the national advisory body, the Indian Nursing Council (Ministry of Health and Family Welfare 2005, 57). Even so, the state level Nursing Councils who are responsible for the accreditation and inspection of training institutions continue to endorse training institutions that do not meet the required standards (Evans, Razia, and Cook 2013, 2).

Critical medical anthropology approaches have highlighted how "the medical hierarchy replicates the class, racial/ethnic, and gender hierarchy" (Baer, Singer, and Susser 2013, 52). Historically in India, the profession of nursing has been highly gendered, with women still making up the vast majority of the workforce. The profession has also been highly stigmatized due to work-related practices and tasks that are seen as culturally taboo for women. These include having to "work outside the home (including at night), to touch strangers, to mix with men, and to deal with bodily fluids (considered polluting within Hindu and Muslim cosmology)" (Evans, Razia, and Cook 2013, 2). As such, traditional caste-based labor divisions have meant that most nurses have been lower caste Hindus and Christians.

Many hospital administrators expressed concern about the distinction between the roles of nurses in India, compared to that in developed nations. Dr Rao explained this as "a different cultural attitude," noting "in the West, the nurse is a decision maker. Here a nurse is a person who follows orders. The way she presents herself or projects herself is not what a medical tourist is probably looking at."

Several doctors and hospital administrators also discussed how the low status of nursing in India is representative of both social and cultural attitudes, many of which derive from a broader gender bias that exists in the wider community and reinforced within the medical community in India. This was highlighted in a conversation with Dr Desai, where he noted "our post-operative care is not that good and that is why in the West the turnaround is better, because the nursing care is better." Dr Rao noted that the specific sociocultural perception of nurses as low status is fostered through nurse education and training and then reinforced in the workplace. This was an issue of concern for senior staff at his hospital as they viewed it as a barrier to "internationalizing" their services and the "world-class" treatment they aimed to provide, and promote, at the hospital.

In a proactive attempt to shift this perception, Ramrakhyani Hospital introduced a range of measures to bridge the "gap" between this imaginary of international medical tourist expectations and the status quo in nursing clinical practice and competence. The hospital ran a nursing college located across the road from the main building, but also developed an intensive induction program and on the job training for incoming nurses, intending to retain nurses within the hospital. The development of the hospital's nurse training program was not born from altruistic or social justice motives to improve the status of nurses, but instead, as Dr Rao explained, it was to ensure "that [nurses] can function profitably in the way that we want them to function."

Key elements of the hospital induction program for their nurses included English, deportment, and grooming classes conducted by external consultants from the airline industry. Dr Rao explained that these classes were an effort to "internationalize" their nursing workforce. Their use of consultants from the airline industry for grooming and deportment classes speaks to the image and branding aspirations of the hospital (as examined in Chapter Three). What Dr Rao was inferring was that they have incorporated their labor force into their branding efforts; in this case, the hospital's international branding.

Many international airlines have traditionally focused their branding on in-flight glamour, of which their highly polished cabin crews play a significant role. As such, airline cabin crews often undergo strict grooming and deportment training prior to commencement. One former attendant from Singapore Airlines described the instruction and rules set during her 15-week training program, which included the setting of specific hairstyles, make-up, and acceptable nail polish colors (Halfpenny 2019). As detailed in Chapter Two, commodification of a health service's labor (in this case the nurses) is one of the factors that demonstrate hypercommodification of the sector.

Further, the statement makes explicit the patient base of the hospital, or at least those they are marketing to. English is widely spoken across Mumbai, but it is the language of the elite: business people, professionals, and the upper and upwardly mobile middle classes. Thus, their *local* service base is the elite. There is a further assertion that their international patients are English speakers, signifying the specific international patients they are targeting (i.e., Westerners from English speaking nations such as the United Kingdom and the United States).

THE INTERNATIONAL MOBILITY OF
MEDICAL PROFESSIONALS

Internationally, the mobility of the medical workforce has steadily increased both in relation to where they are educated and where they work. The medical workforce shifts in and out of different scapes, driven by international and local logics of power that territorialize, de-territorialize, and re-territorialize the workforce. This has serious implications for healthcare systems and, ultimately, population health outcomes for nations. Medical tourism is one of many factors that contribute toward the direction of these flows in the medical workforce. As noted in Chapter Three, the international mobility of the medical workforce is employed as a branding mechanism to attract high fee paying domestic patients and international patients alike to the Indian tertiary healthcare sector. The marketing and branding of consultant surgeons as internationally trained, both by their institutions and themselves, forms part of the affective work in expressing legitimacy and gaining trust of both international and high socioeconomic local residents. This similarly applies to the hospitals with regard to their affiliations with international medical brokers, international accreditations and affiliations with university medical faculties in the United States.

Indian health professionals are acutely aware of the status afforded to international health experiences and qualifications, specifically when undertaken in developed nations. There is additional status and employment value associated with experience attained in OECD countries including the United States, Canada, the United Kingdom, Australia, and New Zealand.

In 2013, there were over 155,000 Indian students studying abroad in six countries (see figure 5.2). In 2010–2011, approximately 12% of all student visas granted in Australia were from India. This number had dropped from the year before when they accounted for 20% of all visas granted (Australian Bureau of Statistics 2012). It was reported in 2014 that over 50,000 Indian students were enrolled in educational institutions across Australia. Paradoxically, many doctors working in the sector expressed that they thought it was still possible to get a high-quality medical education in India, but outcomes were better guaranteed for those that are educated overseas.

The global shortage of healthcare workers and their inequitable distribution across nation-states has drawn significant critique during recent decades. Key concerns have centered on the postcolonial and ethical implications related to the exodus of qualified healthcare professionals from developing nations to developed countries, sometimes referred to as the South–North "brain drain." The shortages within the skilled healthcare workforce are one of India's most intractable problems for the healthcare system and health outcomes of the nation, with at least 6.4 million additional healthcare workers needed

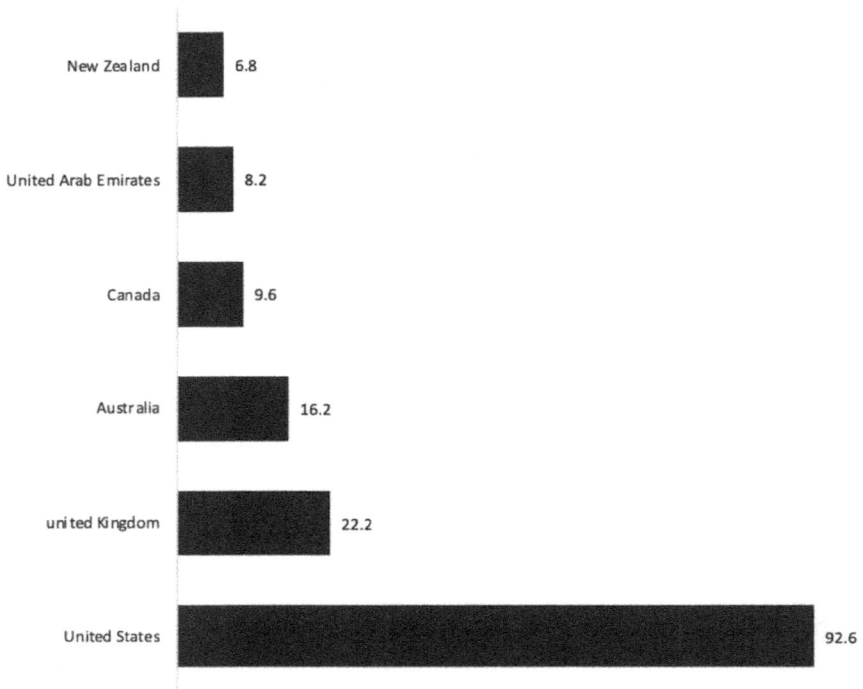

Figure 5.2   Indian Students Enrolled in Tertiary Studies Abroad (Thousands). *Source*: Image created by author. Data from UNESCO Institute for Statistics (2014).

even meet the minimum recommended ratio for the ever growing population (KPMG 2016).

Many OECD countries have become reliant on overseas-born doctors for their health workforces. For example, in 2011, 48% of doctors in Australia were foreign born, with 2,625 Indian doctors migrating to the nation between 2006 and 2011 (Siyam and Dal Poz 2014). Similarly, although the population of the United States is approximately one quarter the size of India's, the number of physicians registered in each nation is similar (United States, 916,000; India, 936,000) (Ministry of Statistics and Programme Implementation 2013; Young et al. 2011). Given this inequitable distribution of doctors, it is perhaps even more concerning that over 50,000 Indian medical graduates are practicing in the United States (Duttagupta 2011). Further, the Global Association of Physicians of Indian Origin has reported that there are about 1.2 million Indian doctors practicing medicine in countries outside of India (2016). This equates to more Indian doctors working outside of the country than within.

In 2010, the WHO adopted a code of practice on the international recruitment of health personnel with the aim to manage the global flow of workers more equitably (World Health Organization 2010). Although intended as a legislative instrument, the code is voluntary and nonbinding for signatory states. One study reported that the code has had minimal impact on the recruitment policy, regulation, or practice for developed nations with the highest intake of skilled foreign healthcare workers (Edge and Hoffman 2013).

One of the arguments employed to promote the benefits of medical tourism in developing nations is that the phenomenon will serve to stem the external flow of healthcare professionals internationally (Mullan 2006). There is speculation that the flow of health workers out of India is easing, particularly with the growth of local corporate tertiary health institutions. This transition has been underway for several decades, corresponding with wider trends of health professionals returning to Asia from OECD nations. Ong and Collier have noted that this return of skilled workers represents "one of the largest repatriations of global skills in recent times" (Ong and Collier 2005, 31), a sentiment regularly echoed by informants in this study. By example, Dr Patel, a senior cardiologist, described the shifting residential patterns of Indian doctors, where although many still choose to study internationally, they return to India to live, "You will see some trends changing in that most of the doctors that used to be living here, they go abroad, they take education, they settle down there. Nowadays they are not settling down there. They take their training abroad, and they come back."

Others stipulated that the changes to the global mobility of health workers away from India is yet to materialize, with Dr Rao, another senior administrator stating, "until such time as we are able to match up their skills [to jobs], both nurses and doctors will go abroad." An opinion piece published in The Hindu concurred, reporting that although some health workers do return to India, this was only a small percentage of those who leave and is mainly health workers in the latter years of their careers. Indian students undergoing training abroad have good reason to stay on in their country of training after the completion of their degrees due to "Better salaries and facilities abroad, easier access to research funds, working on cutting-edge topics and many others are part of the mix" (Altbach 2014, n.p.).

The comparative salaries in different nations impacts on national price setting of healthcare services and is a major determinant of transnational medical tourism flows. Hence, the low global cost of medical services in India is directly related to the low salaries paid to workers in the sector. The significant difference in average annual wages for typical healthcare professionals in the United States and India are illustrated in figure 5.3. The salaries paid in India range between one-third and one-fifth lower than that in the United States (see figure 5.3). This data accounts for international exchange rate differentials, representing the respective purchasing power parity ($PPP) salaries.

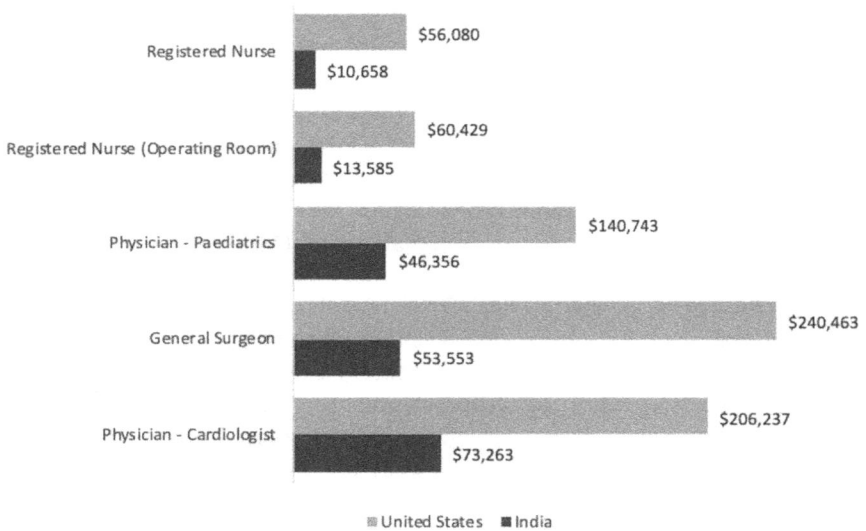

Figure 5.3   Median Salaries for Selected Healthcare Professionals in India and the United States (PPP$). *Source*: From World Bank (2014).

The impact of the long-term and short-term losses of qualified health workers from India, particularly from the perspective of the public health system, manifests in several ways, including the depletion of public investment in subsidies toward the education of the workers, and reduces the quantity and quality of the workforce. Informants also discussed other factors influencing the mobility of doctors and patients, referring to the flow of poorly trained doctors out of India to nations where there is greater demand and capacity to pay higher salaries.

Discussing why some of his patients from the Middle East and East Africa come to get treated in India, Dr D'Costa explained that it was primarily related to their perception of the poor quality of their doctors at home, noting "In East Africa they don't have the expertise and in the Middle East they don't trust the doctors and the surgeons. They are undertrained or badly trained. The Middle East is a dumping ground for doctors who are badly trained."

Another closely related issue is the practice of surgeons and specialists conducting short-term travel to other nations to undertake specialized surgeries, engage in training and research, and to boost their international profile. From Dr D'Costa's perspective, this is a practice that predates the new forms of patient travel, "Some of [the doctors] come here from overseas to operate. I know many German doctors who come here twice a year, make a considerable sum of money and then go back. It's been happening for a long time."

Indian doctors also routinely engage in clinical tourism outside of the country to perform treatments as well. One of the informants in the study explained that there are increasing numbers of fly-in-fly-out (FIFO) surgeons from India who travel to Dubai for short periods to conduct surgeries for multiple patients in between their regular practice in India. Several studies have indicated that the unprecedented growth of the private sector has led to the appropriation of health workers from the public system. Even though health professionals are being trained at much higher rates than ever before, there are still critical shortages of health workers, doctors, and specialists across all levels of the healthcare system, in both rural and urban areas. The National Council on Macroeconomics and Health found that by the mid-1990s approximately 75% of specialists in the country were located in the private sector (Ministry of Health and Family Welfare 2005).

INTERNAL MOBILITY OF HEALTH PROFESSIONALS

Several studies have indicated that the unprecedented growth of the private sector has led to the appropriation of health workers from the public system. Even though health professionals are trained at significantly higher rates than ever before, there are still critical shortages of health workers, doctors, and specialists across all levels of the public healthcare system, in both rural and urban areas. The National Council on Macroeconomics and Health found that by the mid-1990s approximately 75% of specialists in the country were located in the private sector (Ministry of Health and Family Welfare 2005). A study by Rao and others (2011, 590) reported that over 80% of medical physicians are employed in the Indian private sector, driven by poor salaries and working conditions in the public sector. Another study of perceptions of medical tourism by Indian physicians in tertiary hospitals by Qadeer and Reddy (2013) also identified the economic incentives of the private sector as key to the shortage of doctors in the public system. Further, the majority of healthcare investment is centralized in tertiary healthcare, accounting for 80% of the market share (Bajaj 2021).

Another significant issue of internal brain drain is that the majority of tertiary institutions under development in the private sector are built in the urban centers of the nation. The significance of this uneven sectoral distribution is further highlighted by the extreme shortages of specialists in public Community Health Centers (CHC) across India, ranging from 92 in Tamil Nadu through to 990 in Gujarat. On average, 40% of public Sub Centers (SC) function without any health workers, offsetting any apparent or realistic value to communities. Although public Primary Health Centers (PHCs) have lower human resource problems across the major states, there are still several states where over 20% of PHCs operate without doctors (Ministry of Health and Family Welfare 2005).

THE IMPACT OF MARKET-LED HEALTHCARE ON PROFESSIONAL MEDICAL ETHICAL STANDARDS

The Indian healthcare industry's capacity to improve the quality of care across the tertiary sector is severely hindered by widespread corruption, in both public and private domains. Healthcare corruption is driven directly by medical professionals, operating within the context of weak regulatory and monitoring regimes (Anand 2003; Fochsen, Deshpande, and Thorson 2006; Ravindran 2008; Thomas and Varghese 2010; Jhala and Jhala 2012; Mazumdar 2014). The lack of regulatory oversight to enforce or monitor service delivery is particularly problematic in the tertiary sector. Further, medical professionals receive very little professional medical ethics training, with the "exercise" of swearing in MBBS graduates to the Hippocratic oath waning to the point of fatigue (Pai and Pandya 2010; Jhala 2012; Mazumdar 2014).

The Medical Council of India's code of ethics is outlined in the *Indian Medical Council (Professional Conduct, Etiquette and Ethics) Regulation 2002* (hence referred to as The Code of Ethics). The Code of Ethics details the ethical duties and responsibilities of medical doctors, including that relating to their character, practice, quality assurance, conduct, and payment for their service. In particular, s.1.8 notes, "the personal financial interests of a physician should not conflict with the medical interests of patients." (Indian Medical Council 2002, 2) Transparency International have ranked India as the 30th most corrupt country in the world, with health ranking as the second most corrupt sector (after the police force). A quarter of the respondents in a household survey reported having paid a bribe for healthcare services, with the majority of the bribes paid to hospital staff to access hospital services. The report claims that individual doctors and hospital workers drive corruption in the sector (Transparency International 2006).

A significant characteristic that emerged from the ethnographic research informing this book related to the significant differences between the motives, ideologies, and professional medical ethics of a "younger," commercialized generation of doctors compared to the "older" generation of pre-SAP trained doctors in India. The older generation of pre-SAP doctors regularly discussed their work and profession in the context of philanthropy and their service to the vulnerable within the nation. By contrast, conversations with younger post-SAP doctors were more regularly aligned with a preoccupation of larger macroeconomic processes of the nation, how they as doctors could promote their careers and establish themselves better in the local and international healthcare marketplace. Mazumdar (2014), in an article on healthcare ethics in India, similarly identifies the "fearful tendency among many fresh medical graduates. They are ignorant of the ethical basis of medical practice" (2014, 412).

Dr Nayar, an exemplary example of the older generation of doctors in the city, had been working in the healthcare industry from an early age. During initial meetings with him, I asked him what his interests were in his life and work. He frankly and sincerely replied, "Everything." Dr Nayar would rise every day at four in the morning, meditate, complete his daily household chores, read and eat breakfast before leaving his apartment in a small, upper wing of the hospital. He always presented at his office by seven and worked until around seven in the evening. He had a wide range of external interests including playing the sitar, cricket, writing poetry, and learning in general. He explained that learning more about the world around him was his passion, demonstrated by his multiple university degrees, certificates, and diplomas.

Dr Nayar's educational background included an MBBS, a bachelor's degree in law, a master's degree in law, diplomas in psychology, hospital administration, industrial relations, and naturopathy, a post-graduate diploma in medical law and ethics, and a certificate in Psychiatry and Psychosexual Medicine. He had also practiced medicine in a number of other Indian states and internationally early in his career, although he had spent the past two decades working at Ganapathiraju Hospital. Dr Nayar held strong social justice and humanist convictions that strongly informed his medical practice. Whenever he spoke of Ganapathiraju Hospital, it was clear that his overriding priority was that of providing healthcare services to the poor. To further his philanthropic vision, Dr Nayar had volunteered as a visiting member of faculty at numerous universities and teaching colleges, held multiple directorial and Chair positions at national health associations, and was an honorary member of the Rotary club.

Dr Mehta, another example of the older generation of pre-SAP doctors in the city, was a busy consultant surgeon who spent most of his time operating in the older, smaller charitable hospitals of the city; those that serviced the lower socioeconomic sectors of the population. In one discussion with Dr Mehta, between his scheduled surgeries, I hurried along beside him and asked if he was concerned about being paid less for his work in the smaller hospitals than consultants in the larger private hospitals. He explained "we don't earn much, but we get more patients, more complicated cases." On average, Dr Mehta worked 14-hour days, moving between multiple hospitals to conduct surgeries. He was unable to rely on the smaller private hospitals to provide the surgical tools he needed because "money is either not utilized properly or they are taken away," so he always carried a briefcase containing his own personal surgical tools with him. Although he undertook some work within the larger hospitals in the private sector, this was not his priority. Dr Mehta was of the opinion that there were not enough experienced surgeons willing to do the work he was doing in the less profitable, charitable arm of the private sector. Another senior surgeon, Dr Patel, described that although he mainly consulted from more prestigious hospitals, he also chose to consult out of Sacred Heart Hospital as a form of "giving back" to his community.

Many of these doctors were well established in their fields of clinical expertise, with decades of experience and had strong, influential medical networks across the city. However, for early and middle career doctors entering and traversing the highly marketized Indian tertiary healthcare system, their success was ever more dependent on their ability to drive business: to develop a profitable and financially viable business operation, predominantly via their ability to attract high profit patients. Many of these younger doctors described the increasing vulnerability of the medical workforce in relation to their profitability. Dr Malik explained that "doctors have to generate practice and they have to generate income for the hospital. If I'm not, then the hospital says I'm not needed any more for my services." Here lies the conundrum for many doctors, their Code of Conduct dictates that they should not expressly solicit clients, yet their employment depends on their willingness and ability to do so.

Dr D'Costa, a senior consultant with over three decades of experience working in a variety of hospitals explained that professional ethical standards had undergone significant changes in recent decades. He noted "a lot of us have got used to a sliding door of ethical standards." Dr D'Costa explained that in India, unlike many nations, financial disclosure was not required nor expected from doctors. For example, the practice of pharmaceutical sponsorship of doctors in India was common and accepted in the sector. He further noted that in other nations he had worked, such as the United States, if a doctor was directly sponsored by a pharmaceutical company, they "would be dragged to the highest ethical boards, and he'd be chastised. In India, we'd be thinking nothing of [it]" and "at the end of the day, anything goes." This is despite specific sections of the Code of Ethics ("Indian Medical Council (Professional Conduct, Etiquette and Ethics) (Amendment) Regulations, 2009 - Part-I) prohibiting any such activities.

Dr D'Costa's assertions that professional medical ethical standards in India have declined in recent decades, aligns with the ongoing commercialization of the healthcare sector post the introduction of the SAPs by the IMF and World Bank in the early 1990s. Examples of medical doctors acting on commercial interests in a manner that violates medical ethical standards are commonly reported in the media. For example, in 2012, a Parliamentary Standing Committee on Health investigated the approval of multiple pharmaceutical products through the Drug Controller General of India on the basis of "scientific" endorsements written by the pharmaceutical companies and on the recommendation of senior Indian doctors. The main contention made in the final report of the Standing Committee was that "(t)here is sufficient evidence on record to conclude that there is a collusive nexus between drug manufacturers, some functionaries of CDSCO [Central Drugs Standard Control Organisation] and some medical experts," further stating that the actions of the medical experts involved were "clearly unethical and may be in violation of the Code of Ethics of the Medical Council of India applicable to doctors" (Rajya Sabha Secretariat 2012, 20). Specifically, the medical experts in question breached the 2009 amendment to The Code of Ethics, which sets out the rules related to relationships between doctors and pharmaceutical companies. This amendment was originally introduced to discourage unethical pharmaceutical sales and marketing by doctors. However, as this case highlights, the Medical Council of India have limited ability to enforce their regulations, relying instead on doctors to self-regulate.

Scheper-Hughes' (2000, 2002a, 2002b, 2003) ethnographic study of transplant tourism, which incorporated fieldwork in India, further addressed the "medical professional corruption" of doctors. Scheper-Hughes addressed the complicity of doctors as actors in networks of organized crime in the illegal trade of organs from living human donors. She too argued that market-led health has weakened the professional ethic and practice of doctors, noting "the conflict between non-malfeasance ('do no harm') and beneficence (the moral duty to perform good acts) is increasingly resolved in favor of the libertarian and consumer-oriented principle" (2004, 62). The engagement of doctors in medical tourism in India further highlights the medical professional corruption referred to by Scheper-Hughes. Medical tourism, from the perspective of doctors, is market-led, consumer and economically driven. Doctors know that treating and attracting medical tourists increases hospital profitability, hence their employability, their income and status in the sector. As such, the medical tourism industry is antithetical to key areas of The Code of Ethics. For example, the incentive for healthcare institutions and doctors to engage in medical tourism is primarily for financial gain, yet section 1.1.2 of The Code of Ethics sets out that "The prime object of the medical profession is to render service to humanity; reward or financial gain is a subordinate consideration." Given the overarching privatized, and commercialized context of the Indian healthcare system, it is difficult to fathom how this rule could abided by at all.

THE COMPORTMENT OF "BIG-MEN" AND
THEIR HIERARCHICAL DOMAINS

In the following section, I present two case study examples from my field-work to describe the manifestations of the hierarchical structures and high levels of competition among doctors and medical administrators for power status, job security, and career development in Mumbai's hospitals. From the time of my initial interviews, I became aware of the significance of these hierarchies in the private medical patronage system of the tertiary health-care sector for myself as a researcher and, more importantly, for the tertiary healthcare workforce. In the first case study, I describe a day of fieldwork in Tayyib hospital that revealed much about the internal culture and political power structure of the hospital. In the second case study, I describe one of the more powerful CEOs participating in the study, Colonel Nandal, outlining his bombastic military style of management and how this shaped his ethical comportment and the hospital's governance. Mines and Gourishankar (1990) have outlined some of the characteristics of "big-man" leadership in India, arguing that in contrast to the big-man of Melanesia, Indian big-men are usu-ally institutionally embedded, and that "such men attract followers and enact their roles as generous leaders through the 'charitable' institutions that they control" (1990, 762). The Colonel was a "big-man" of the city, well known for the medical "modernization" of his hospital and his brashness in publicly refusing to comply with the Bombay Public Trust Act requirement of reserv-ing 20% of beds for the disadvantaged (outlined in Chapter Five).

Case Study 1: The Medical Director, the CEO,
and Medical Patronage at Tayyib Hospital

My first interview at Tayyib hospital was with one of the hospital's Administrative Medical Officers, Dr Chopra. She was a trained medical doc-tor working in the marketing division of the hospital. This level of the hospi-tal was much less opulent than the upper floors that I had viewed on an earlier guided tour of the medical tourist facilities of the hospital. The doctor arrived and ushered me through the doors into what looked like a call center, with small, partitioned offices. Adjacent to her office were several "closed-door" offices, including the hospital's Medical Director. The marketing depart-ment's proximity to the Medical Director's office was spatially revealing, highlighting the growing prominence of business administration processes to the operation of the clinical aspects of the hospital.

I was in a rush, as I was running late for my morning of scheduled inter-views due to, in combination, my daughter's nanny arriving late and par-ticularly bad traffic exiting Chembur that morning. Around 20 minutes into the interview, the Medical Director appeared from his office and walked past with an entourage of five junior Hospital Administrators. The Medical Director slowed when he saw me talking to Dr Chopra. He approached us and began sharply questioning her. The Medical Director summoned Dr Chopra to go with him. After a short time, Dr Chopra returned, quite anxious, and explained that the Medical Director had not been informed of my presence and was extremely unhappy that I was there.

During the next few hours, I was shuffled in and out of multiple levels, areas, and offices within the hospital by numerous people and intensely questioned regarding my credentials and research. I had all of my identity documents taken from me. The CEO, who had granted my entrée to the hospital, was away on business and the Medical Director was infuriated that he knew nothing of what I was doing in his hospital.

Eventually I was told that I was to be removed. Within minutes, two security guards armed with rifles arrived and grabbed my arms to "escort" me out of the hospital. By this time, I was distressed, finding myself carted back down another corridor, up another set of stairs, and across an area I did not recognize. Before I knew what was happening, I had been escorted off the property and was left standing on the street, disoriented.

When I eventually spoke to my primary informant that evening, he was not overly surprised. Although he had not mentioned it before, he explained that there were ongoing "personality problems" between the CEO of the hospital and the Medical Director. The following day, I had a phone call from another doctor under the direction of the CEO, apologizing for the "misunderstandings" and inviting me back to the hospital the next week.

The fury displayed by the Medical Director regarding my presence in the hospital that day revealed more about the everyday practices of power exercised through the medical patronage network in the hospitals and the broader tertiary sector than it did any particular concern he held about the research. From the perspective of the Medical Director, I was present under the patronage of the CEO, who was a rival to his own power and influence within the hospital. As such, I represented a threat for several reasons. First, the CEO had invited me to the hospital, facilitated through his internal medical faction. This had not been communicated to the Medical Director. Further, it emerged that the majority of the prearranged interviewees were within the CEOs faction, which (if nothing else) probably annoyed him. Also, the CEO had strong ties with my medical patron (another influential Medical Director of another major hospital), and they were part of an external medical network that he was not aligned with. Last, although the Medical Director had instructed his own factional staff to remove me after an initial encounter, I was still present in the hospital hours later when he came upon me with Dr Taher, who had set up the interviews.

The failure of his factional staff to have me removed and the defiance implied by my ongoing presence, facilitated by those in the CEO's faction, would likely have caused further aggravation. For doctors and hospital administrators, competition for employment and career trajectories hinge on their ability to negotiate these hierarchical networks of power.

As noted earlier, many doctors wishing to progress their careers seek further qualifications such as the Master of Hospital Administration. Alliances with powerful individuals in the sector are important and influential to safeguard their current and future employability. Those at the top of the hierarchy, such as CEOs and Medical Directors, dictate the conditions for those who work under them, but are also in fierce competition with one another. With the rise of formalized corporate governance in hospitals, the role of CEO has surpassed the authority and influence held by a Medical Director. The younger generations of doctors are acutely aware of this. Dr Lulla, a 35-year-old Assistant General Manager with an MBBS and postgraduate degrees in public health and hospital administration, was adamant that he had no interest in becoming a Medical Director. He had his sights firmly set on becoming a hospital CEO.

Although I was not drawn into the web of power negotiations to such magnitude in other hospitals, I was nevertheless constantly aware that these underlying struggles for influence, authority and control, forming part of the daily life of individual healthcare professionals in the city, were ever present. Neoliberal structures within the quasi-corporate environments of the Trust hospitals facilitate the globalization of their patient base with the rise of medical tourism, viewed as a vehicle from which to increase their income. However, the competitive environment it fosters for those working in the sector is at an intensity that is changing the trajectory of the career-paths of medical professionals. It was no longer enough to attain a medical degree or a specialization in a particular field to maintain employment or progress in the sector. Business degrees, including hospital administration, were increasingly viewed as the only way to progress in "the business."

Case Study 2: Colonel Nandal and His Military-Style Operations at Khalsa Hospital

As described in the Introduction, I relied heavily on the insights of my primary informant and mentor, Dr Nayar, to determine the hospitals that would be most appropriate to situate the fieldwork for the study. As Dr Nayar was intimately tied to the healthcare networks in the city (and nation), he provided me with a list of email and phone contacts of the "big men" in hospitals he thought would potentially accommodate my research needs. He also advised that it would be very useful to include in my communications that I was associated with TISS and himself (rather than stress my association with the University of Melbourne). I took this advice from an early stage but felt very uncomfortable using what I perceived to be "name-dropping" as a technique to negotiate access to the field.

However, as I progressed with gaining access to different hospitals, I discovered it was an essential part of the process. Any mention I might make of the city's "big men" of the healthcare sector created an immediate positive change to the many gatekeepers' receptivity of potential participation in the research. Colonel Nandal, the CEO of Khalsa Hospital, was one such "big man" of the healthcare sector in the city. When others discovered that I had met with the Colonel, it opened doors elsewhere.

Khalsa Hospital was one of the most well-known, multispecialty hospitals in the city of Mumbai. It was established in 1973 and had 359 beds. I spent the least amount of time in this hospital, as the Colonel was relatively skeptical about the premise and methods I was utilizing for my research. Although he agreed to meet with me for an interview, he was less than eager for me to "mill around" the hospital conducting observations. He also let me know that he thought there was nothing that anyone else in the hospital could tell me that he didn't know himself.

The hospital, and the CEO himself, had recently attracted negative media attention with regard to the hospital's noncompliance in treating the required percentage of Scheduled Caste/Scheduled Tribe (SC/ST) patients, also known as the "indigent sector," and he had been admonished for being discourteous to the Legislative Council after being summonsed to appear. Khalsa hospital was one of the hospitals using more open and aggressive marketing tactics to attract medical tourists and approximately 20% of their patients were identified as medical tourists in 2009.

When I first walked into Khalsa Hospital, I found it very difficult to imagine any newly arrived medical tourist feeling at ease in the hospital. The interior and exterior of the hospital were undergoing significant renovations in 2009 and the whole of the front lobby area was in the process of being refurbished, although this was not immediately obvious to the uninformed observer. Granted there were workmen roaming about with building materials, but there were no cordoned off areas with work in progress signs or other safety alerts. This type of scene was not unfamiliar for public hospitals and smaller private nursing homes but felt out of place for an elite private hospital that was well known as a hub of international medical tourism in India. The hospital itself was located in one of the richer areas of the city, situated toward the top of the hill on the bustling street. Half a block up from the hospital was the start of a string of clinics, including an upmarket dental clinic advertising cosmetic dentistry and a family doctor's surgery. Across the road from the hospital was a very large and well-known cosmetic surgery clinic that also has a successful line of very expensive skin treatments and cosmetics.

I entered the building, making my way through the building works, and approached the hospital's reception. The receptionist summoned a security guard and directed him to take me to see the Colonel. I was led to an overcrowded lift and squeezed in alongside the security guard. The security guard led me to an office full of people waiting, with a window-partitioned office at the back of the room. From there, an administration assistant led me to a boardroom further down the hall, one of the few air-conditioned spaces. The walls of the room were lined with portraits of the Hospital Trustees, the founder, and past heads of the hospital. After some time, the same woman who brought me to the boardroom walked me to the office of the Colonel.

The Colonel, a large man, peered over at me from behind a long, opulent, antique desk and requested that I take a seat. His presence was imposing, one likely honed during the 25 years he had served in the Indian Army prior to his appointment at the hospital. The Colonel was born in Pakistan (formerly Sindh) several years before India's Independence and partition from Pakistan. After obtaining a bachelor's degree in political science and history, he had joined the army. Notably, there was a significant presence of ex-military personnel occupying senior roles in the major private hospitals in Mumbai. At the time of our interview, Colonel Nandal had been the CEO of Khalsa Hospital for 15 years and was also the President of the city's Association of Hospitals.

In different media reports published during the time of my fieldwork he was invariably labeled a "man of honor," a "healthcare pioneer," and a "medical technology revolutionary." The Colonel initially attributed his shift from the military to hospital management to his wife, who was the daughter of one of the Hospital's Trustees. He explained that he had discovered that there was very little opportunity for further advancement of his career in the army. The Colonel's explanation of the hospital and his personal background was filled with colorful military descriptors denoting his personal upward trajectory to the lofty height of his position as CEO of the hospital:

> I came here by default. Otherwise, well, it was no use getting silly and lying on the ground. In the army, you attack when there is fire. When they fire on enemy in defense, the enemy is busy with fire, [and] the second line of fire attacks from here: there is no need getting silly and lying down on the ground. I was a pilot, I was a tank man, I was a skydiver, and an off-lander, I'm from tank activity. So, can you see the link? I just got this opportunity by default.

The Colonel explained the formative impact that his time in the military had on him personally, and also how he drew on his military experience to enact power within the management of the hospital:

[I went] from my childhood straight into my old age because my youth went into my uniform. I'm totally disciplined now. I can't leave my old life. I was so used to the army way of functioning. I passed orders and orders were carried out. Then when I came to the hospital, if I passed an order, it would generate discussion. So, the easiest answer we had, I found out, was to just sack everybody on the management. Then I all brought in experts: intelligence officers, naval officers and so on. By the end of the first year, my Medical Director was also an ex-Colonel. The Chief of Pathology is also a retired ex-Colonel. We all speak the same language.

(Colonel Nandal)

The Colonel's reference to bringing in "experts" from the military is indicative of his individual leadership style and the hierarchical governance structure he had developed in the hospital. The time I spent with Colonel Nandal revealed his bombastic comportment, whether discussing his background or current pursuits. His explanation of how he improved the financial position of the hospital is indicative of this style:

I am not a healthcare man, and I happened to meet the Board of Trustees. When they gave me a chance, this hospital was quite in the red. Totally no equipment was working, strikes by the union and so forth. I told them to give me a chance. Now I have a totally debt free hospital. I have crores of surplus, I have equipped the hospital, my hospital is the best hospital. The best equipments in the whole country. When I first arrived, everything was new to me, I did not even know what a catheter is. But now, if there is a man dying, there is no heart surgeon available, I will do the heart surgery.

(Colonel Nandal)

It is worth noting that the Colonel did not have a medical degree, nor any form of medical training. He further explained that he continued to maintain his authority at the institution by removing anyone that questioned his decisions. He rationalized this by asserting that it was one of the reasons he was able to "turn the hospital around," returning it to fiscal stability. However, in the year before I met the Colonel, a delegation from the Maharashtra Legislative Council had visited Khalsa hospital to request the patient records of the hospital to determine whether the hospital was complying with charitable hospital regulations that require one-fifth of all patients to be treated free of cost, as designated by cultural and socioeconomic status. In a show of his big-man status, and likely noncompliance of the hospital, the Colonel refused the delegation access to the hospital data.

Hansen (2005) has argued that actions such as this typify the "Indian middle-class world," where there is a contempt for the rules and an "expectation of being able to 'fix things' by pulling a few strings, or by merely asserting one's importance" (2005, 169). The Colonel, nonetheless, was later publicly admonished for his actions. However, local identities, such as the Colonel, were instrumental to the construction of what Whiteford (2000) has labeled "idioms of hope." Explaining the different localized experiences of health commodification in Cuba and the Dominican Republic in the 1990s, she argued that although health commodification may be driven by global economic and political forces, it is "internalized in local idioms and identities." Whiteford extended the notion to explain that "Global processes are played out in the cultural, historical, and political contexts in which they occur, and they have distinct consequences for the presentation and experience of health" (2000, 59).

The local idioms of hope extended by many of the doctors and managerial staff centered on perceptions of the growth of, and their participation in, the development of this new order of "world-class" services, equipment, and treatment at any of their respective hospitals. Embedded in notions of modernity, and India's ascendence and place in the world order, medical tourism verified these idioms of hope for the health workers via a myriad of aspects.

VIEWS OF THE MEDICAL TOURIST: CASH COWS, RECIPIENTS OF GLOBAL PHILANTHROPY, OR EVIDENCE OF WORLD-SYSTEM ASCENDENCE?

Healthcare workers extended a range of views related to their perceptions of the medical tourists they treated from individual, institutional, and national perspectives. There were three intersecting views commonly referred to, all of which were highly dependent on the medical tourist's global region of origin. First, medical tourists were often framed as a vehicle to advance their careers, their hospitals, and the healthcare system at large. Medical tourists, particularly those originating from wealthier Western nations, were viewed as bringing in much needed financial capital to support and maintain their consultancies, justifying their place at their respective hospitals and demonstrating their global specialist status. Further, the profit derived from medical tourists was cast in relation to the facilitation of philanthropic services at the hospitals.

A second framing was the view of medical tourists as "medical refugees" and their work in providing healthcare services to these medical tourists performed a philanthropic function in alignment with other forms of development aid. This aligns with literature depicting particular forms medical tourism as medical exile (Inhorn and Patrizio 2009; Kangas 2010; Ormond and Lunt 2020). Medical tourists framed in this manner by health professionals were generally from regional countries such as Bangladesh and other countries in the Global South.

Third, medical tourists were viewed as evidence that India was indeed emerging as a global leader in healthcare, ascending the world order to that of "world-class" nation. The Colonel, and many other doctors and hospital administrators, expressed great satisfaction regarding the growth of medical tourism in India. The notion that people from other nations, particularly from the global North, would undertake transnational travel to access services in their hospitals was a matter of both national and great personal pride. One of the Colonel's strongest passions related to his leadership was his role in modernizing the institution by bringing the most up-to-date biotechnologies to the hospital. Ong and Collier have argued that for many Asian nations, biotechnologies "are allied to nationalist efforts to overcome past humiliations and to restore national identity and political ambition" (Ong and Collier 2005, 3). In a similar manner, the doctors and hospital administrators consistently reminded me that they were working in, and helping to develop and shape cutting edge, world-leading tertiary institutions. Informants always discussed the "world-class," "international standards," and frameworks employed in their hospitals. In doing so, they actively pointed to the changing status of India as a developing nation and their individual or collective agency in bringing about this shift. Dr D'Costa described how tangible shifts related to globalization, transnational flows of people, and the status of India as a country in the world-system were already well underway:

So that person from the US . . . would come here, the streets would be crowded with people watching you go by because they'd say, "gosh we'd never seen a person like this." Many of our relatives fled India to migrate anywhere else in the world, and we thought we were the unlucky ones to be left behind. I am amazed that people from all over the world have come and live in Mumbai. We have Americans, we have Italians, we have Germans, we have French, all kinds of people from all over. Even Australia, I mean, you've come to live in Mumbai. So, it shows how things have changed so much.

Most doctors and senior hospital managers were also eager to discuss their own extensive international travels and international qualifications. The Colonel regaled me with stories of his own travels internationally during the past year for medical conferences, holidays and more. The day following our interview, he told me, he was due to fly to Hong Kong for a conference, followed by Frankfurt, Munich, Tel Aviv, and finally the United States.

Most doctors I spoke to would introduce the issue of "remaining in India" early in our conversations. They wanted to make sure I understood it was his or her intentional choice to work in India and not in a developed country. This

Table 5.1 Healthcare Personnel Shortages in Selected Indian States

Selected Major States	Sub Centres (2004)		Primary Health Centres (2004)		Community Health Centres (2004)	
	Population per SC	*No health workers (%)*	*Population per PHC*	*No doctors (%)*	*Population per CHC*	*Shortfall of Specialists**
Kerala	6,250	25.6	34,125	2.0	276,861	342
Tamil Nadu	7,154	–	45,008	0.0	1,774,600	92
Andhra Pradesh	6,048	51.0	50,824	6.2	470,360	432
Maharashtra	9,947	10.0	54,355	0.9	253,277	429
Karnataka	6,476	60.8	31,408	0.0	209,262	325
Gujarat	6,956	25.6	47,287	20.7	186,705	990
West Bengal	7,746	33.5	68,390	15.6	844,432	247
Punjab	8,516	31.2	50,184	13.4	207,598	238
Haryana	8,665	–	51,674	0.0	292,819	239
Assam	5,214	97.8	43,669	0.0	266,380	–
Bihar	8,018	–	50,291	–	820,584	–
Madhya Pradesh	6,835	17.4	50,574	21.2	266,013	867
Orissa	6,193	–	28,633	3.8	158,905	–
Rajasthan	5,689	27.2	33,715	7.8	189,507	723
Uttar Pradesh	8,939	69.1	45,619	–	564,806	–

Source: Ministry of Health & Family Welfare (2005).

was demonstrated in an observation made by Dr D'Costa, who explained his experience returning to India after practicing in the United States, noting "when I trained in the US and came back, people thought that there was something wrong with me, that perhaps I'd done something wrong to have to come back here."

Underpinning many of these conversations was an assumption that working in India might be perceived by others as a personal failure, implying a lack of choice or lower level of skill or acclaim. By reframing themselves as active agents in a choice making process, and "world-leaders" in the political and economic transformation of the nation, the doctors were defending their professionalism, while reconstructing their social identity from that of powerlessness to one of power. Further, given the high levels of unqualified physicians practicing within the nation, their assertions were also an affirmation that they were not one of "those" doctors.

CONCLUSION

This chapter described the internalization of the processes of hypercommodification for the local medical workforce in Mumbai, addressing the significance of different forms of mobility of healthcare workers, the interchanges and flows of people, power, and knowledge systems. As such, the new mobilities and reconfigurations of the medical workforce regarding where they train and practice, along with how they see themselves, their futures, and the healthcare system is paramount to both the fledgling industry, but also to India's healthcare system. This mobility and internationalization of the skillset of Indian doctors is indicative of market fluctuation, with international supply and demand of health professionals remaining of high import.

The rapid hypercommodification and marketization of the sector has created a highly competitive environment for those in the local workforce. The vulnerability of workers in the sector can be illustrated by the turnover of staff in the years following my fieldwork. Medical directors, CEOs, and upper level administrators have been removed, retired, or replaced by up-and-coming hospital administrators, many headhunted from the corporate sector. However, the rising tide of international medical tourists traveling to their hospitals in the city of Mumbai has also inspired nationalistic and professional pride in local tertiary healthcare workers. Embedded in these feelings of pride is a transformed social and medical imaginary of India's shifting status in the world system, and their facilitating role as providers of "world-class" care.

This chapter has addressed how the different forms of engagement by healthcare professionals with ideological representations of health and healthcare are transforming the sector, particularly in terms of the logics and practices of the healthcare workforce. Significant changes have been experienced in approaches to education, training, professionalization, credentialing and standardization of the personnel in the hospitals I studied, which are all critical to understanding the medical tourism industry in India.

Chapter 6

The Structural Violence
of Medical Tourism

Gated Enclaves and Health Exclusion

Medical tourism is aligned with increasing flows of geographic and economic mobility for some and is directly connected to the immobility of others. It supports and reinforces barriers to a wide range of goods and services for local host populations, contributing to the deterioration of health equity in the nation. As such, this chapter focuses on the impact of the structural changes engendered and propelled by medical tourism for the largely impoverished local populace of Mumbai. What of their experiences during India's race to invest in and build a new order of "world-class" super-hospitals to capture foreign exchange from international patients? What have been the wider effects of the hyper-commodification of tertiary healthcare and concurrent disinvestment in public healthcare? For example, how has this population fared with the privatized reconfiguration of healthcare services during the global COVID-19 pandemic?

These questions are addressed by tracing some of the lesser explored pathways and footprints of medical tourism across the city of Mumbai, locating the vertical links that connect it to broader local inequities experienced within the population. By doing so, the chapter further problematizes key arguments related to the promotion of medical tourism, focusing on the local social, cultural, and structural conditions in which the industry operates. It illustrates how medical tourism supports and reinforces the economic and geographic stratification of the wider populace, driving inequity in access to tertiary healthcare services, whilst also shifting the resource focus away from primary healthcare.

MEDICAL TOURISM, GLOBAL AND
POPULATION HEALTH

There have been few nuanced examinations of the impact of medical tourism for either global or population health in scholarly debates. Global health, from an epidemiological standpoint, has been defined as the focus on health issues "whose causes or redress lie outside of the capability of any one nation state" (Taylor 2018). Global health approaches generally centralize the importance of improving health outcomes and achieving health equity for all people internationally. Similarly, population health refers to the health outcomes, and equitable distribution of outcomes, amongst a group of individuals (Kindig and Stoddart 2003). Both concepts are framed by social justice principles and are underpinned by the notion that the functioning of all societies is highly dependent on the health of its members. Further, both concepts support the proposition that health inequity, poverty and social injustice are inextricably linked as determinants of poor health.

Most simply defined, inequity refers to "an unfair and remediable inequality" (Feachem 2000, 1). Health inequity is then the relative disparity in health status between different subgroups of a population. The concept of equity necessitates a moral and ethical dimension, focusing on "creating equal opportunities for health and with bringing health differentials down to the lowest level possible" (Whitehead 1991, 221). Although equity approaches to health are broad in scope, many question the different mechanisms and approaches to the distribution of healthcare services across populations. This is highly pertinent to medical tourism, particularly in contexts such as India, where the industry plays a role in informing the direction of national healthcare policy, resource allocation, and infrastructure expansion.

As already described in earlier chapters, medical tourism is an industry that focuses on technologically advanced, highly specialized healthcare services, specifically targeting international patients with a greater capacity to pay for these services than the vast majority of the resident population. That is not to say that medical tourists themselves are a homogenous group of wealthy global citizens. To the contrary, as detailed by many scholars of medical tourism, medical tourists are heterogenous groups with diverse social, political, and economic capital who engage in the practice for diverse reasons (Kangas 2007; Song 2010; Crooks et al. 2010; Horton and Cole 2011; Inhorn 2011; Solomon 2011; Ormond 2015; Speier 2016; Whittaker and Leng 2016). However the freedom[1] of individuals to engage in medical tourism infers a relative global socioeconomic status that enables this specific form of transnational mobility.

The urban configurations, in which the sites of medical tourism are located, including hospitals, accommodation, and other services, reveal stark inequities in the distribution of health services to different populations in Mumbai, and India more broadly. Medical tourists are the consumers of Mumbai's "luxury" health services, whilst the majority *Mumbaikars* have little access to any services at all. The opportunity to traverse international borders in the pursuit of health is not possible for most of the world's population and is definitely out of reach for most of Mumbai's residents. As noted by Roberts and Scheper-Hughes (2011, 7), "the ability to travel and the status it embodies" is significant. This tension between heterogenous mobile and immobile populations draws noteworthy attention to the significant global inequities accentuated by medical tourism. Whittaker and Leng (2016) have proposed that in response to the decline of state responsibility for the provision of healthcare and consequent privatization of services, medical tourism embodies an emergent flexible biocitizenship enacted by the heterogenous groups engaging in medical tourism. In this conceptualization, Whittaker and Leng build on Ong's (1999) theory of flexible citizenship. In this theorization, mobile medical tourists are cast as active agents and transformers of biocitizenship. Yet this framing of active transnational flexible biocitizens does not address those with less flexible biocitizenship, including the vast immobile populations depicted in Greene's legal immobility theory of poverty (2019). So, how do we extend this theory to analyze the impact of flexible biocitizenship on these immobile populations across the globe who are so often the host populations of medical tourism?

To recast our focus to the host populations of medical tourism, theories of critical tourism studies are highly productive to explicitly examine not only the tourist, but the impact of tourism on the hosts and the ecosystems that sustain the activity. Caton and others (2018, xxi) explain that through the lens of critical tourism studies, tourism is understood as "a complex sociocultural practice with equally complex consequences for destination places and for the collective and individual lives of both hosts and guests." However, the extant literature on medical tourism has paid scant attention to the multifaceted consequences it holds for the individual and collectives in different contexts. Gupta and Ferguson (1997, 6) have argued that in the past, "anthropological approaches to the relation between 'the local' and something that lies beyond it (regional, national, international, global) have taken the local as given, without asking how perceptions of locality and community are discursively and historically constructed." Gupta and Ferguson (1997) extend this contention, noting that many frame "the local" as the static, natural, authentic base that is intruded upon by the new, modern, and artificial "global."

By tracing the figurative footprints of medical tourism across Mumbai, this Chapter seeks to embed and contextualize its central thesis that the industry and practice leads to greater inequities in access to healthcare for host populations, reinforcing and driving disruptions to the healthcare system, the institutions in which it is located and the workforce delivering the services.

This is undertaken by examining the consequences of medical tourism to the dynamic ecosystem, including the sociopolitical and cultural structures, of which medical tourism in Mumbai is embedded. The urban configurations of the sites of medical tourism, including hospitals, accommodation, and other services, reveal stark inequities in the delivery of health services to different populations in Mumbai.

POPULATION HEALTH IN MUMBAI

Across India, it is estimated that more than 100 million people live in urban slums (Ministry of Housing and Urban Poverty Alleviation 2011). There is very little data collected and reported on that captures the inter and intra slum variabilities, leading to the likely underreporting of many health outcomes and little understanding of how these populations navigate India's complex healthcare system to access services. In a study of slum residents in 13 slums located in Mumbai, it was reported that the majority of households earned less than USD 180 per month (lower than the national minimum wage) and the most common occupations of the residents (predominantly men) were as drivers, shop/stall attendants or owners, tailors, and household assistants (Naydenova et al. 2018).

The majority of women (83%) were engaged in unpaid labor in the home. Less than half of all participants had ever had their blood pressure or sugar tested and most with noncommunicable health conditions had never taken targeted medication. Most pregnant women had accessed basic maternal services but nearly 80% of women in the study thought that maternal healthcare was too expensive and nearly three quarters reported their access to care was hindered by distance. Importantly, it was found that the vast majority of participants favored private providers, despite the greater expenses incurred, due to perceptions of these services being safer and of greater quality. Private healthcare providers were most frequently accessed by participants for all conditions, with the exception of maternal health. However, the private sector referred to were mainly private primary healthcare providers located within the slum communities.

SOCIO-SPATIAL DETERMINANTS OF HEALTH IN MUMBAI: ON THE WRONG SIDE OF THE FENCE

The Greater city of Mumbai is the capital city of the state of Maharashtra and the commercial hub of India. Alternatively labeled the "City of Gold" or "City of Dreams," the Mumbai of Bollywood and popular culture is littered with clichéd images of what Indian journalist Mayank Shekhar colorfully refers to as:

A city of the underworld, guns, bar and the item girl; the beautiful hero, his heroine and the songs they make love to; the rich bourgeois and his skyline; the slumboy, the starlet and the millions they could still make: a mythical, maximum city of the active mind, and colonial-gothic architecture. (Shekhar 2011, n.p.)

The city is home to over 20 million residents and is the most densely populated urban agglomeration in the India and the fourth highest in the world (Government of India 2011b). With such a tightly compressed populace, more than half of the city's population live in the *jhopadpattis* that extend across and envelop all corners of the city. More than 40% of the residents of the city of Mumbai live below the national poverty line (United Nations Development Program 2010). Given the vast socioeconomic divides experienced across the city and nation, it is worth noting that India has experienced high levels of economic development during the last half century. However, the uneven distribution of its dividend has compounded many of the wider population's health, education, and socioeconomic status.

In 2000, the nation's President of the time, Dr K.R. Narayan, gave his most celebrated address, outlining his perception of the greatest challenges facing the country:

Fifty years into our life in the republic we find that justice—social, economic, and political—remains an unrealized dream for millions of our fellow citizens. The benefits of our economic growth are yet to reach them. We have one of the world's largest number of illiterates; the world's largest middle class, but also the largest number of people below the poverty line, and the largest number of children suffering from malnutrition. Our giant factories rise out of squalor; our satellites shoot up from the midst of the hovels of the poor...The unabashed, vulgar indulgence in conspicuous consumption by the nouveau riche has left the underclass seething in frustration. One half of our society guzzles aerated beverages while the other has to make do with palmfuls of muddied water. Our three-way fast-lane of liberalization, privatization and globalization must provide safe pedestrian crossings for unempowered India also so that it too can move towards "equality of status and opportunity." (Narayan 2011, 145–46)

Over two decades later, much of Narayan's speech remains pertinent to the "wicked" problems faced by India. The gap between the rich and the poor has widened with Basole (2014) reporting that inequality had increased beyond that of the colonial period by the end of the 1990s, inclusive of social, gender, and cultural inequality. Gupta (2012), among others, have questioned the waning political focus on inequality, outlining the structural violence of the fragmented and arbitrary local bureaucratic processes in India that operate in indifference to the experiences of those most disempowered.

At the beginning of the twentieth century, 25 million people, or 10.8% of India's population resided in urban areas. By the turn of the 21st century, the urban population of India had grown to 286.1 million, almost 30% of the total population of the nation (United Nations Development Program 2009; World Health Organization 2009). Projections estimate that by 2030, the urban population will grow to over 550 million people (Bhagat and Mohanty 2009, 7) and that the urban population will overtake the rural population of the country by 2045. This ongoing demographic transition has, and will continue to have, a significant impact on population health and the delivery of healthcare services in India.

Mumbai and New Delhi are both included in the top ten most populous cities of the world (United Nations 2018). In Mumbai, the population has grown exponentially from the time of the country's Independence and is the seventh most populous city in the world. Although the city's geographic boundaries have expanded alongside the population, this has not occurred at the same rate. Consequently, population density is extremely high, with an average rate of 24,000 people per square kilometer (Government of India 2011) and the price of land has climbed sharply.

The 2010 Mumbai Human Development Report noted that "Housing is so exorbitantly priced that even the middle-class tends to move into hutch-like apartments, into tenements whose size precede only slums—*chawls*" (United Nations Development Program 2010, 38). The UN-Habitat defines slum households as those residing in urban areas that lack one or more of: durable, permanent housing; no more than three people sharing a room; easy access to affordable water; access to sanitation; and tenure security (UN-Habitat 2018).

The Indian census estimated that the city of Mumbai had over one million slum settlements that housed 41.3% of the city's residents (Government of India 2011). This ratio decreased by about 10% over a decade, but in real terms it shifted from 5.8 million in 2001 to 5.2 million in 2011 (Government of India 2006, 2011). The western suburbs of the city also have much larger slum populations than the rest of the city, with the highest ratio in the Mankhurd-Govandi area where 95% of the population reside in slums (Deshmukh 2013, 34). Other estimates suggest that a further 10% of the city's population is homeless, or "pavement dwellers" (Appadurai 2000).

It is in this context that elite private hospitals in the city engaging in medical tourism now form a part of networked precincts of privilege, sometimes referred to as "gated communities," appropriating vast tracts of highly sought-after land in impenetrable zones of socioeconomic spatial exclusion. The phenomenon of constructed, infrastructure-rich, and safe urban havens, available only to the relatively wealthy, infiltrates multiple spheres of social life. What began as gated residential complexes and shopping mall precincts expanded to the gating of entire neighborhoods in different areas of the city. These gated zones are promoted as areas of respite and luxury for the upper middle classes of the city, represented as an escape from the poverty-stricken city-dwellers, in enclaves of luxury, elitism and conspicuous wealth, prosperity, and consumption.

Although the urban Indian middle class are highly heterogeneous, there is a specific socially constructed segment that Mathur (2010) has categorized as a "New Middle Class." The "New Middle Class" share an upward social mobility, high levels of education and salary, and emerging patterns of consumption practices similar to those identified in the United States, where "access to selected commodities, brands and services has become a means for securing upward social mobility and virtually upgrading one's position in society" (Mathur 2010, 213). The New Middle Class include many of the doctors and health administrators focused on in this book.

These microcosms of social exclusion and exclusivity across the metropolis of Mumbai take many forms, including the conspicuous gated suburbs, townships, and clusters of high-rise apartments. The gating of these zones is predominantly physical, with walls or fences enclosing set areas. The fences or perimeters are guarded by armed watchmen that patrol the premises around the clock to ensure that only those "allowed" can come and go. The gated communities in Mumbai and other urban capitals across the nation are demonstrative of a social transformation that began in the early 1990s, particularly in the metropolitan centers. Importantly, this form of geospatial stratification coincided with the implementation of neoliberal policies earlier described (i.e. the NEP and the conditionalities set out in the World Bank and International Monetary Fund's SAPs).

The significance of gated communities to this study became apparent soon after my arrival in the city in 2009. In the first instance, as a newly arrived "Westerner," I was directly ensconced in the gated environment of the University community at the Tata Institute of Social Sciences (TISS). Similar to many other universities internationally, the TISS campus was scattered across a large area on the outskirts of the city. Many of the university staff (academic, professional, and service) reside on-campus in small, low-rise apartments. Located on the fringes of the city, the campus is lush and green, backing on to a large, forested area. After several weeks living on-campus, I moved into a leased external apartment, about a kilometer away from the University. The apartment was located in a gated cluster of four high-rise apartments. Within the bounds of the gated society buildings there was a clubhouse, a gymnasium, a large swimming pool, and a 750-meter walking track around regularly maintained, manicured gardens. The perimeter of the property was fenced, serving as a barrier to entry for the larger populace.

The residents of the society buildings were mostly couples or small families, mainly high-caste Brahmins working in professional roles, falling within Mathur's categorization of India's New Middle Class. Most families had one or more servants of lower caste Hindu or Muslim background. Many servants were "live-in" and were primarily young and female. Although there is strict regulation forbidding child labor, it is widely disregarded in the employment of household labor. In part, these gated islands serve to re-establish, reaffirm, and reinforce the hierarchical social and cultural divisions that have operated in India for centuries. Caldeira's (2000) ethnographic account of São Paulo evoked similar depictions of a "city of walls" that form barriers to protect the rich and keep out the poor.

The exclusivity related to inclusion within a community, and exclusionary measures keeping "others" out, are expressly marketed as aspirational features of residences in gated communities. One advertisement of apartments in a set of "Society Buildings" in Mumbai in 2009, featured the title "Take a coronation" with an image of a Victorian era armchair and accompanying text, "Not for everyone," evoking the high imperialism of a colonial palace and associated exclusion. This can be understood as a form of affective marketing to the elite of the city and nation. Hospitals engaging in medical tourism employ similar strategies, using affective boosterism to attract medical tourists and elite locals, with reference to signature standards of luxury they offered.

Medical tourism operates within the context of this fortification and stratification of the upper middle-class, high-caste population from poorer, lower class and caste residents. Upon entry to India, medical tourists are bustled through airports into luxury cars and whisked across the city into five-star hotels and/or the hospital equivalent, often in gated neighborhoods. These forms of inclusion and exclusion created by urban gating can also be productively viewed through the lens of the "worlding" of cities, such as that theorized by Roy and Ong (2011). In Roy and Ong's edited collection, the authors argue that the "worlding city" is a both a site of emergence and a "mass dream," where the term "world-class city" is wielded as a "talisman" by politician and urban elites alike to justify specific projects and redevelopments. Chapters focusing on India explore how the idea of "world-class city" has been used invariably as a means to dispossess the poor of their land in Bangalore (Goldman 2011), clear slums in Delhi (Ghertner 2011), or in rearticulations of a Global Indian city in Kolkata (Roy 2011).

In Mumbai, the local spatial politics of the city are historically associated with its growth, its largesse and place as the financial hub of the nation. It is situated on the west coast of India and was formerly made up of seven different islands, which over the course of five centuries, were gradually connected by land reclamation projects to form what was known as the city of Bombay. In 1995, the name was changed to Mumbai, representing the Hindu Goddess *Mumbadevi*, the patron goddess of the Kolis (fisherfolk) and Agris (salt collectors), traditional inhabitants of the seven islands that form the contemporary megacity of Mumbai. As noted by A. Gupta and Ferguson (1997, 6), "anthropological approaches to the relation between 'the local' and something that lies beyond it (regional, national, international, global) have taken the local as given, without asking how perceptions of locality and community are discursively and historically constructed."

Gupta and Ferguson extend this contention by arguing that many frame "the local" as the static, natural, authentic base that is intruded upon by the new, modern, and artificial "global." The local importance of place, belonging, and social hierarchy in the city of Mumbai was always contested and fluid during conversations I had with *Mumbaikars* from all walks of life. On one particularly long taxi ride back to my apartment in Govandi after a day of archival research in Colaba. I engaged in a lengthy discussion with the taxi driver. He told me his story of how he came to be living in Mumbai driving taxis. He was born in Kashmir to a reasonably wealthy family and consequently was well educated and politically informed. However, over his lifetime, his family gradually lost their money through their "investment in the wars of Kashmir." As a result, he decided to leave his family to come to Mumbai in search of work. Unemployment rates are exceedingly high in Kashmir and have been increasing.

The Kashmir region is made up of two states, Kashmir and Jammu, and is located at the northern tip of India. The region shares common borders with both Pakistan and Afghanistan. It has a Muslim majority, compared to the Hindu dominance in the rest of India, but had been ruled by Hindu Maharajas for a century leading up to the partition of India and Pakistan in 1947. The region has been caught in an ongoing territorial tug-of-war from the time of Partition, with both nations making claims over the states, leading to three official wars between the two countries over the dispute. In more recent years, there have been increasing internal calls for the independence of the region from both India and Pakistan. Curious about his thoughts on these matters, I asked the taxi driver his opinion of the call for Kashmir's sovereignty. Despite the highly volatile history, he casually replied that he didn't care too much, as Mumbai was now his home. I had incorrectly assumed that given his background, he would be pro the state's independence and actively invested in the outcomes of the region. Instead, he went on to tell me about his progression in Mumbai from rickshaw driver to the highly coveted taxi driver-owner position he held today. He spoke proudly of how he had been living in a chawl just outside of Colaba for four years, after initially living in the jhopadpattis.

Our conversation turned to the housing problems in Mumbai, and how the already dire overcrowding was accelerating due the constant influx of people into the city. It was at this point that he began to vehemently expound that there should be state laws in place to prevent more people from coming to Mumbai, as there was simply no more room. He had very little empathy for those seeking work in the city from other areas, despite his own relatively recent migration. He was not the first, nor last, person I encountered with such passionate views on the topic of the growth of the city. On a separate occasion, a rapid escalation during an exchange with a different taxi driver led me to fear I would be hurled from his cab, or worse, when he declared that I "should not be allowed in the city" as I, an outsider, was taking up space that Marathis could be occupying.

This issue of the ever-growing population of the city through immigration from other states of India is referred to in a key preferential policy platform of the Shiv Sena. The Shiv Sena vigorously promotes the ideology of "Maharashtra for the Marathis." This platform is primarily directed toward South Indian migrants, where the Shiv Sena promotes the notion that they steal jobs that "rightfully" belong to Marathis. The platform is also driven along religious lines, with Hindu nationalism bubbling at its core, similar to the long-held political manifesto of Prime Minister Narendra Modi.

Another account signifying the importance of social belonging and community cohesion in Mumbai occurred shortly after my arrival to the city. On this occasion, I was walking through Deonar from my apartment building to the TISS. After passing by a large group of auto-wallahs, standing around smoking cigarettes and sipping chai in the muggy heat, I approached the busy corner; the intersection of a road that crosses the Thane River to Navi Mumbai. As I walked closer, I noticed a man lying on the ground, lying in a large pool of his own drying vomit. It seemed likely that he had been there for some time. In alarm, I looked down to the group of auto-wallahs, wondering why they were not doing anything. The group of men gave no indication of any interest in the man whatsoever. I ran down the busier road hoping to find someone to come to the man's aid.

Within several minutes I encountered a police officer and explained the scenario. The police officer shot me a look of incredulity and stated, "nothing to do madam, nothing to do." Thinking the policeman may not have understood, I reiterated the situation, to which he retorted "What to do? Really madam, nothing to do," going further to explain that the man, whether dead or dying, must be a "no good person." His rationale was that if the man was a "good person," the auto-wallahs would have assisted him, as the community in the area was very cohesive and knew who "belonged" and who didn't, or who had been cast out for "bad behaviors." He noted that it was evident that there would be just cause for the lack of action toward the man. The policeman then explained that even if he wanted to, he wouldn't be able to find a doctor who would agree to come and see the man, as they would want to know how they would get paid. "What about an ambulance?" I asked. However, similarly, ambulances were predominantly owned by the private hospital sector, so it was still an issue of "no money, no action."

Later that evening, after returning to my apartment, I discussed the scenario with an acquaintance. Her view of the situation was similar to that of the police officer. She also concluded that he must be a "bad man," outside of the community structures that protected "their own." The health of the majority of residents of Mumbai is highly dependent on access to healthcare services, which are determined in large part by their sociocultural and socioeconomic status.

The high rates of early mortality and morbidity detailed in the data (see Chapter Two) can be readily observed across the city in the prevalence of street beggars with amputated limbs pulling themselves along uneven pavements on carts, the women with decimated, burnt, and scarred faces and bodies from being set alight by in-laws seeking dowry revenge, and the small, desperately undernourished homeless children running in groups in the railway stations. The meager resources allocated to the public health system provide no social safety nets in Mumbai large enough to support the sheer mass of people eking out an existence in such circumstances. People rely instead on their family, kin, and patronage networks to ensure their safety, their health, and in many cases, their survival. Within this context, the logic of market-led healthcare is confounding, and hypercommodification of the healthcare system nothing short of absurd. Regardless of the growing demand for healthcare within the local population, medical tourism builds the fences around hospitals ever higher; while the rapidly widening gaps of socioeconomic inequity dig the trenches ever wider to further fortify the hospitals.

CONNECTING SOCIAL INEQUITY TO LOCAL HEALTH INEQUITY

The Nobel Award-winning Indian economist and philosopher, Amartya Sen (2001) argues that development efforts of nations should be focused on attaining human freedoms for societies as both the end and means of development. There are particular freedoms that are necessary for Sen's version of development: political freedoms; transparency in social relations; freedom of opportunity; and freedom from abject poverty. These freedoms are inclusive of "both the processes that allow freedom of actions and decisions, and the actual opportunities that people have, given their personal and social circumstances" (A. Sen 2001, 17). He argues that the sign of true human progress—or development—is the enhancement of all four freedoms and that a nation's development is indicated by the free agency of its people. As such, Sen's understanding of poverty is vastly different to income-based measures, viewing it instead as the level of capability deprivation for an individual. Sen theorized that a person's capability matters instrumentally, as any individual may only achieve the substantive freedoms they have the agency to attain. He further highlighted the importance of factors such as age, gender, and social roles to capability. Many of the local structural conditions in Mumbai, namely the abject poverty experienced by many, are inherent barriers to the freedoms articulated by Sen (2001).

There were many formal and informal slums surrounding the apartment I lived in during fieldwork. One study has estimated that 95% of the population of Govandi lives in slum dwellings (Deshmukh 2013). I would wander through these areas on most days to shop for fruit and vegetables, and to catch the train, taxis, or auto-rickshaws. These slums are a mixture of *kachcha* and *pukka* residences. The *kachcha* housing is usually erected on and around building sites where the workers would create their own spaces to live while working. During my time in Mumbai, I visited the residence of two young women that worked for me as maids. The two women had been hired by my landlord to clean my apartment on a daily basis as part of a nonoptional segment of the lease. Their home was located in one of the older, established, legal slums in Deonar. Many of the residences in this particular *jhopadpatti* are semi-*pukka* housing, in that they are made from more solid, longstanding materials compared to the mud, cardboard, and blue plastic tarpaulin constructions found in many other areas.

The buildings were dual-level, two-roomed residences, attached to one another in long winding laneways. Although some have electricity connections, these are unregulated, makeshift, likely hazardous, and commonly siphoned via illegal means from nearby power mainlines. In spite of this, many of residences in this *jhopadpattis* had televisions and access to cable network television. However, the infrastructure in the slums is poor, with low levels of sanitation and access to water. In most of these areas, the only toilets available are small blocks that cater to thousands of residents.

The health implications of the poor infrastructure were never more apparent than during the monsoon season. At the onset of the season, I was puzzled by the sudden inconsistent attendance of the young women to my apartment. After several weeks of intermittent arrivals, I discussed the matter with the younger sister. She told me that all of their family had been ill and that this regularly occurred during the monsoon season. The conversation then turned to the extra individual work burden that came as a consequence of the illnesses in the family. On top of her regular duties, she now also had to collect the family's daily water provisions from the tap located at the far end of the slum in place of her ill sister. Every day she carried a large earthen pot to the tap at around five in the morning, wait for an hour in line for her turn and then carry it back home on her head. I asked her if she boiled their water before using it as a general practice, as I was aware the waterways of the city were often contaminated during monsoon flooding.

One study found that water contamination and low levels of sanitation cause infections and disease that account for around 40% of the total mortality in Mumbai slums (McFarlane 2012). The younger sister explained that they never boiled their water and thought it an odd suggestion, despite their daily practice of boiling the milk delivered to *my* door and meticulously filling a dozen water bottles with water from the water filter installed in the kitchen. Health literacy, along with general literacy, remains very low for the residents of slums in India. This is particularly the case in the megacities of the nation, highlighted by multiple studies of slums in Mumbai and other urban centers of the country (Bapat and Agarwal 2003; Chaplin 1999; Graham, Desai, and McFarlane 2013; Karn and Harada 2002; Yesudian 1999). She also told me that it was common for their employers (of whom they had multiple in the apartment blocks within which I lived) not to pay them when they were away due to illness. However, it was also a common and expected practice that employers, as patrons, contribute to medical expenses for their household employees.

By comparison, one of my acquaintances, Magdu, lived in *kachcha* housing in one of the colonies north of Govandi and had always boiled her water, as she was taught to do so at Catholic boarding school in Pune, where she was raised. However, she too had to rise at six every morning to fill two large water drums and carry them back to her apartment before boiling them. Although this acquaintance and her family tended to avoid monsoonal sickness, she often suffered from serious migraines yet would rarely see a doctor for their treatment. Instead, she would ask friends, family (and myself) what medicine they took for headaches. Based on these recommendations, Magdu would buy whichever medicine she felt the most fitting from one of the many street-front chemists. At these small street-side stalls, there were no requirements for prescriptions for any pharmaceutical product. If you had the money, and had the product, they would sell it to you. One street vendor told me that an "American" would come to him once a year to buy boxes and boxes of generic branded Viagra to take them back to the United States to sell. He said he sometimes had other foreigners buy large quantities of Valium to take back to sell in their countries of origin as well. On one occasion in Ramrakhyani Hospital, an older Indian woman who resided in the United States, explained to me that whenever she came home to India to visit family, she always accessed general "check-up" services in the hospital, and would "stock up" on all of the medication she and her family in the United States needed as they were so much cheaper, and of "better quality."

One day Magdu came to visit me with a friend to request my opinion regarding a medical matter. Magdu, had decided, despite my protests that because I was researching an issue that was health related, that I must know about medicine. Magdu's friend was five and a half months pregnant and did not want to keep the child. Both women knew it was possible to get some "pills" from the chemist that would terminate a pregnancy and had procured a box of mifepristone, a widely used drug for inducing labor, earlier that day. Mifepristone is not recommended for women past 12 weeks of pregnancy, but neither woman was aware of this.

The pregnant woman had planned on taking it immediately, but Magdu had decided they should come and see her "doctor friend" to see what I had to say. Given she was far past 12 weeks in her pregnancy, the consequences of taking the drug could have induced a range of life threatening complications. I shared this information with Magdu's friend, explaining the high risks involved and advising her to seek advice from a medical doctor. Although not entirely impressed with the information provided, Magdu's friend thankfully decided not to take the mifepristone and the two women took leave to seek assistance elsewhere. The pregnant woman was not overly receptive to seeking maternal health services in the public sector as she was of the opinion that these services were of low quality, but she said that she knew of reasonably priced private providers located close to her residence. As noted earlier in in reference to the study of Mumbai slums, maternal healthcare is one of the few services reported to be relatively accessible in Mumbai (Naydenova et al. 2018).

Examples such as those outlined in this section highlight how local social and cultural issues coupled with individual factors such as low health literacy and poor infrastructure can have disastrous effects on the health of populations in cities such as Mumbai. These factors are further compounded by the difficulty and expense of accessing safe medical treatment compared to the ease of access and lower cost self-treating health problems with pharmaceuticals obtained on the street.

Health equity, similarly to income poverty, should be assessed by accounting for the variety of contextual conditions that impair, maintain, or improve the health of people. The capability deprivations and substantive freedoms that enable or deprive individuals, families, and communities in the different decisions they are capable of making significantly impacts on their health. However, it is also important to note that economic inequities remain a significant determinant of the health of individuals and populations, particularly when there are no public safety nets to offset these factors.

For those unable to pay, the consequences can be dire when serious or chronic illness arises requiring access to tertiary healthcare services. Further, the social opportunities that are provided by society for individuals to access education and healthcare, housing and access to sanitary infrastructure are highly influential for their substantive freedoms. This is because education, healthcare, and adequate housing enable far more than a person's opportunity to live a long and healthy life, but also enable more inclusive and valuable participation in a range of other social, cultural, economic, and political activities. Medical tourism creates and reinforces physical, economic, and systemic barriers to healthcare access for the majority of Mumbai's residents, in a highly effective, multipronged gating of the sector, impinging on more than the health of residents, but their substantive freedoms.

COVID-19: SPOTLIGHTING THE CRUMBLING STRUCTURES OF A HYPERCOMMODIFIED HEALTHCARE SYSTEM

Soon after the emergence of Covid-19 in late 2019, its rapid international transmission led to the WHO declaring it a global health emergency by 30 Jan 2020. As a result, on 25 March 2020, India implemented one of the most stringent lockdowns internationally, limiting the mobility of its approximately 1.4 billion people, with a notice period of only a little over three hours. The most strict phase of the lockdown continued for two months, leaving millions of urban migrant workers homeless and unemployed, exacerbating horizontal inequalities across caste, gender, and religious lines, and (across 2020) pushing upwards of 750 million people into poverty (Gisselquist and Kunda 2020; Jagannathan and Rai 2021; Raman et al. 2021). By early May 2020, India was reporting daily infection rates of Covid-19 of more than 400,000 with a cumulative official total of more than 24 million cases of infection across the nation (Kansal 2021). However, many commentaries noted the likely undercount of these data. Dr Nayar explained to me that this second wave had caught the government and, in turn, those within the healthcare system "by surprise," in that they had vastly underestimated the potential likelihood that such a voraciously infectious second wave of infections would sweep the nation.

Internationally acclaimed Indian author Arundhati Roy (2021) published a scathing piece in The Guardian UK, depicting the Indian government's failure to effectively respond to the Covid pandemic as a "crime against humanity," caused by the "massive privatization of India's healthcare." Roy described the brutal humanitarian crisis unfolding in the nation, including, wards with no staff and more dead patients than live ones. People are dying in hospital corridors, on roads and in their homes. Crematoriums in Delhi have run out of firewood. The forest department has had to give special permission for the felling of city trees. Desperate people are using whatever kindling they can find. Parks and car parks are being turned into cremation grounds. (Roy 2021, para. 9)

Roy addressed the emerging medical markets flourishing in this context, including more obvious markets for medical equipment such as oxygen saturation machines, but also the bribes to facilitate final viewings of family members in hospital mortuaries, fees for priests to deliver final prayers, and corrupt online "medical" practitioners spruiking bogus Covid treatments and remedies. She also noted that the exorbitant fees of private hospitals to access treatment had impoverished families at all ends of the socioeconomic spectrum, where "just the deposit alone, before they even agree to admit you, could set your family back a couple of generations" (Roy 2021, para. 11).

Doctors on the frontline of the COVID-19 response in the public health-care system have reported that although bed capacities have expanded to cope with the extraordinary demand, no additional doctors were engaged to manage the workload. Further, workforce numbers actually declined in many areas given many of the postgraduate students who ostensibly constitute the bulk of the workforce within public hospitals tested positive to the virus (Mehotra and Ghosal 2021). The failure of the government to prioritize the national, and potentially world's largest, vaccination schedule drew equally fierce criticism.

By mid-April 2021, India was recording the highest global daily case rate of new Covid-19 infections, approximately 300,000 a day, with sky-rocketing mortality rates "characterized by the shortage of oxygen supply in hospitals, shortage of vaccines, unavailability of hospital beds, fires, and oxygen leakages in hospitals" (Jagannathan and Rai 2021, 19).

As of June 2021, only 2% of the Indian population was fully vaccinated. The government has invariably blamed the slow rollout on shortages of supply and a variety of structural and technical issues experienced during the process. Multiple technical barriers to vaccination were reported, including the process of accessing a vaccination appointment in the public system. People had to first download a mobile application, register, and book an appointment. However, there were ongoing technical problems barring registration and causing the application to crash. Even when people managed to register and attempt to book appointments, they experienced up to two month wait times. Further, given not all people own mobile phones (20% in in Mumbai slum populations alone (Deshmukh 2013)), and the disproportionate distribution of healthcare services in rural areas, barriers to accessing vaccines are more pronounced.

However, for a nation known as the "pharmacy of the world," supplying somewhere in the range of 20 to 60% of the world's vaccines, the inability to vaccinate its own population during a global pandemic is paradoxical. During an interview in April 2021 for *The Conversation Weekly*, Professor R. Ramakumar (in Merino and Ware 2021) posited that the slow rollout was less a problem of technical barriers, instead the result of a series of significant policy gaffes at a national level. Foremost, the central government's original decision to only access two (Indian produced) vaccines, Covishield and Covaxin, constituted a serious miscalculation of how quickly the vaccines could be produced and delivered to the nearly 1.4 billion people of India. It was only later that the central government amended the scheme to add the Russian Sputnik V vaccine to the national vaccination plan.

In initial central government policy, the government was the sole provider of the vaccines. Only those over the age of 45 were given access to the vaccination free of cost, with all others required to pay between INR 400 and 600 for full vaccination, depending on the vaccine accessed. This policy was unevenly rolled out between states, with some providing the vaccines free to all and others providing no subsidies. In early April 2021, the central government amended its approach to provision, retaining 50% of the supply for the national program, and the remaining 50% shared equally between the states and private providers, thus instigating the deregulation of vaccine pricing, resituating vaccinations within the broader frame of the hypercommodified healthcare system. Facing public backlash, the central government again shifted their vaccination policy in early May, acquiring 75% of all vaccines manufactured, which they then passed on to the states to alleviate the burden of negotiating with manufacturers. Further, Prime Minister Modi declared that all vaccinations would be administered free of cost in the public system from 21 June 2021 (Menon 2021).

The remaining 25% of vaccinations were still available for private procurement, but in a winding back of their earlier deregulation, the government also set caps of INR 780 for all three vaccines (Menon 2021). However, already marketized, the impact of these vaccine caps is yet to be determined. For example, earlier in the year, luxury vaccination packages were offered by corporate hotel chains across the nation. Lalit Hotel Mumbai was reportedly hoarding vaccine vials and offering various vaccine "experiences." Their marketing package "Get Vaccinated & Rest With Us," offered two "experiences" of vaccination, the first priced at INR 3,500, inclusive of a room and set menu meal at the hotel for 3–4 hours, and the second at INR 5,000 including an overnight stay, meals, and Wi-Fi (Mandhani 2021). The uncanny parallel between these vaccination packages and similar medical tourism packages rest in the elite population targeted, privileging their needs over and above the remainder of the population. Social media photos of Bollywood stars receiving their Covid vaccination at the nation's elite hospitals reinforce these notions of the dual-tiered rollout of the vaccines.

An example of such is the photo shared on Instagram by Varun Dhawan at Hospital A, posing against a background printed with the checkered logo of the hospital resembling that of backdrops used for red carpet shots at glitzy film awards nights ('Varun Dhawan receive first dose of Covid-19 vaccine, thanks the 'wonderful doctors'' 2021). Media reports further indicated that a black market for oxygen and vital medicines emerged during 2021, ostensibly driven by a combination of the rapidly escalating case numbers, shortages of medical supplies and inaccessibility of healthcare services for the population (Ellis-Peterson and Rourke 2021). Those with sufficient economic and social capital reportedly started hoarded these medical supplies, leading to even greater supply shortages within many public (and private) healthcare institutions (Yasir 2021), again reinforcing the inequalities experienced within and across the population.

As earlier noted in Chapter Four, from the time the Covid-19 pandemic emerged, the wealth of the nation's richest have continued to grow, whilst staggering proportions of the nation's 1.4 billion people have been driven into crushing poverty. The already significant inequalities evident both across and within most segments the population have widened exponentially. The Covid-19 pandemic has, in turn, hastened the processes of hypercommodification within the healthcare system, resulting in healthcare services for the most disadvantaged more out of reach than ever in a time of unprecedented need.

CONCLUSION

The examples outlined in this chapter reiterate the potentially devastating effects that the ongoing privatization and commodification of the healthcare sector, supported by medical tourism, has for large sectors of the population in Mumbai and across India. Chapters 4 and 5 illustrated how medical tourism, alongside local and external forces of commodification, drives up the cost of healthcare in many of the private charitable institutions that treat the majority local residents of Mumbai and the nation. If these models of healthcare financing continue with such heavy reliance on out-of-pocket household payments, those that will bear the highest burden of these costs are the host population of medical tourism, the residents of the nation. The implications do not go unnoticed by the healthcare providers, who feel both the push and the pull of engaging with the trade. Dr Rao, for example, discussed the stark realities of seeking to increase medical tourism trade for the people of India.

> If I focus a lot on medical tourism obviously, I'll increase my charges. That means my local people, if I don't have a dual billing, will have to pay more. And the infrastructure costs, to match up to international standards, which I feel is required, will increase the costs again, and the local population will not be able to afford it.

The structural, managerial, and pricing shifts underway in hospitals in the city seeking to attract medical tourism directly and indirectly impact on the rates they charge. Although many of the local population will not have ready access to these services, there is extensive evidence detailing how the private sector sets the pricing for both private and public sectors, particularly for tertiary services (Bhat 1999; Duggal 2007; Yesudian 1999). As medical tourism drives prices higher, the more it detrimentally impacts on the vast majority of the host population, where more than one in five people already avoid treatment when sick because of the cost burden (National Sample Survey Organization 2006b).

Medical tourism operates within the context of the fortification and stratification of the upper- and middle-class population from the poorer, lower caste, and class citizens of India. In combination, the ongoing trends of population health inequities, public health funding decline, growing levels of out-of-pocket expenditure, and increasing vulnerability to healthcare prices raise significant questions about the rationale of directing resources toward commercially driven, private healthcare models.

Contributions from government and private industry continue to fortify and encourage medical tourism in developing nations, with claims it has the potential to revive floundering local health systems through stimulating economic development. However, the second you step inside the opulent surrounds of an international patient suite in one of the prestigious "5-star" private hospitals in India, and compare it to the crumbling, overcrowded, open wards of the public hospital only blocks away, it is evident that there are significant gaps between discourses of stimulus and reality.

Beyond the rapid development of these hospitals are local populations facing critical health issues and widening social, cultural, and economic inequities that impact on their access to healthcare. This situation is exacerbated in many of the countries actively promoting medical tourism, where public health funding incrementally decreases while continuing in patterns of healthcare system commodification. If understandings of medical tourism are reframed to focus on the widening inequities within and between local populations, immediate questions arise about the distribution of both benefits and disadvantages that stem from the industry, and the structural violence that medical tourism inflicts on the poor.

Dominant rubric centers on the parties benefitting from an industry that has both public and private entities pouring resources into high-cost, high-tech care for the comparatively rich, inversely to the epidemiological needs of the population. The "comparatively rich" includes the elites and growing middle class of India, alongside those that Milstein and Smith (2006) refer to as the disenfranchised American "medical refugees" without health insurance. The aggressive rush to a new, modernized, world-leading, advanced, and professionalized India implies a tacit acceptance that the "haves" of the world have a greater right to health than the "have nots." When the medical tourism industry is celebrated and promoted in a context in which it remains the norm for the poor to expect to be thrown into crippling debt if illness requiring tertiary treatment strikes, it is, *ipso facto*, a clear and considered form of violence. On this matter, I agree with Gupta's argument that "certain classes of people have a stake in perpetuating a social order in which such extreme suffering is not only tolerated but also taken as normal. All those who benefit from the status quo and do not wish to see it changed then become complicit in this violence against the poor" (Gupta 2012, 21).

Through the lens of a rights- and equity-based framework, this chapter has depicted some of the more detrimental social and health outcomes resulting from the uneven distribution of healthcare for the wider Indian populace, and the role of medical tourism within the related structural hierarchies. The chapter paints a bleak picture of the potential hazards of furthering a market-led agenda for the healthcare system of India, particularly if achieved without addressing and remediating the associated equity impacts.

NOTE

1. In this context, I invoke Sen's (2001) use of the term freedom within a capability framework.

Conclusion

Local Imprints of the International Neoliberalization of Health

The primary focus of this book has been the examination of the variety of impacts of medical tourism for the local hosts of the wider city of Mumbai. That is, what are the localized effects of medical tourism for healthcare institutions, their healthcare workers, and the local population of the city? In doing so, it recasts the lens away from medical tourists themselves, of whom are centralized in much of the extant literature. By following the tracks of the metaphorical elephant of medical tourism, as described in the Introduction, this book has also provided detailed descriptions of local manifestations of medical tourism and its associations with, and implications for, the national healthcare system and local supply chain networks related to the phenomenon. The book has detailed the associations between the patterns of hypercommodification within the Indian healthcare system and the emergence of medical tourism in this context. In this chapter, I highlight the major arguments of the book, further emphasizing how the study adds to understandings of healthcare inequities globally. The chapter further addresses the major theoretical, methodological, and practical implications of this multi-scaled analysis of power relations across different social institutions and actors.

ASSOCIATIONS BETWEEN THE LOCAL HYPERCOMMODIFICATION OF HEALTHCARE AND MEDICAL TOURISM AS A GLOBAL PHENOMENON

In the first section of this book, I introduced the local context of the ethnography, briefly describing the main features of the five hospitals in the study, and the city of Mumbai. I positioned the book in the context of the literature on medical tourism and outlined its relationship to relevant economic development theory, explaining the use of critical medical anthropology and a rights-based approach to the framing of the research, data collection, and analysis. The first two chapters premised the significance of the commodification of healthcare to the growth of medical tourism as a global phenomenon, specifically within India, and how the transition toward a hypercommodified sector has directly impacted on health equity in the nation. I also introduced some of the main factors that led to the global shift toward the commodification of healthcare and healthcare systems, addressing the role of international organizations such as the World Bank and the International Monetary Fund. By comparing and contrasting the Indian healthcare context to that of other key nations promoting medical tourism services, I highlighted the specific problems and vulnerabilities that medical tourism has on health equity in the nation.

THE TOURISM OF MEDICAL TOURISM

The significance and relationship of "tourism" to the phenomenon of medical tourism can be clarified by examining the links between medical travel to cultural circuits of the broader tourism industry. Many of the features of the hospitals where this ethnography was set (re)produce those of Indian luxury hotels, including physical design attributes, development of hospital branding, expansion of services, digital marketing tools and partnerships with third-party facilitators. The development and application of affective branding techniques are evident in hospital architecture, spatial design and experiential space making that aligns with signature hospital brands.

There are pivotal factors that present external barriers to these hospitals success or lack thereof, in attracting international patients. These barriers also replicate those affecting the success of the broader umbrella of tourism, including sudden macroeconomic events, political unrest, and disease outbreaks. This has been demonstrated with clarity during the coronavirus pandemic that has swept the globe since early 2020, with the industry all but grinding to a halt. However, optimistic ideas of the industry's recovery mobilize and (re)surface across the globe as first, second, and progressive waves of infection sweep different nations.

THE QUASI-CORPORATIZATION
OF TRUST HOSPITALS

One of the core dilemmas described in this book is the local manifestations of the impact of the shifting economic structure on tertiary healthcare institutions in India, particularly the disruptions that have been experienced within the not-for-profit sector. Healthcare systems across the globe have shifted toward market-led models, with intensive commodification of services capturing foreign clientele who are attracted to far less expensive services of India and similar economies. It is in this context that many of the financially faltering not-for-profit hospitals have reset their management processes, transforming to corporate structures. For many, these changes have not arisen through choice, but out of necessity to keep the doors open. Philanthropic and religious Trust hospitals in India are usually established with the principal aim of providing services to the lower castes, classes, and other vulnerable sub-populations. With the shifts to corporate management, these philosophical foundations have been replaced by the need to attract more patients who are able to pay more for their services, such as international medical tourists and wealthy locals.

In chapter 4, I traced the history and religious traditions related to philanthropy in India and the role this sector has played in healthcare provision to the wider population. Outlining the recent histories of several Trust hospitals, the chapter also addresses the links between the new corporate governance management styles, increased costs of services, and their reduced capacity to service the needs of disadvantaged groups. Specific historical shifts in the economic and structural conditions of the city have led to the diminished financial viability of Trust hospitals, forcing many to close and others to significantly shift their ethos, governance and financing mechanisms. The particular set of economic structural conditions of India in the late nineties and first decade of the 21st century facilitated the entry of a new class of corporate, for-profit hospitals in the city. The influx of corporate hospitals fostered a highly competitive private healthcare market, which occurred alongside the enduring decline of philanthropic funding directed toward charitable hospitals. Many large charitable hospitals have responded to these conditions by outsourcing their management to corporate companies: some to large corporate hospital networks and others to major industry conglomerates. By doing so, the Trust hospitals experienced a rapid shift toward market-led practice and governance, transitioning to a new form of quasi-corporate hospital. The most immediate impact of these changes for local residents was an inflated cost structure of their tertiary healthcare services. The price increases can be traced back to corresponding upgrades to infrastructure, standardization processes undertaken to satisfy national and international accreditation requirements, integration of advanced biotechnology, and "add-on" hospitality services. Many of these "upgrades" are also closely associated with the intent of hospitals to attract higher paying, international medical tourists. Although different hospitals have had additional contextual factors that have led to their quasi-corporate transitions, the outcomes for patients are the same.

Many of these large Trust hospitals have historically played a prominent role in providing services and care to the poor in Mumbai. Although there are regulations in place stipulating Trust institutions reserve a percentage of their bed capacity for the most disadvantaged groups, these rules are rarely enforced by authorities and are regularly contravened. The lack of capacity within the city's public hospitals to provide sufficient services to cater to the majority of the resident population, coupled with the declining interest of quasi-corporate charitable hospitals, portends dire outcomes for many local and regional residents.

MEDICAL TOURISM AND THE HEALTHCARE WORKFORCE

From the early 1990s, significant shifts emerged within the Indian tertiary healthcare workforce in relation to their increasing mobility, the development of professional standards, and the impact of the marketization of healthcare on their daily practice and professional ethics. In chapter 5, I argued that these changes have contributed to an environment that is highly competitive and fiercely hierarchical for the healthcare workforce. The growing hyper-commodification of the sector is driving generational changes in the attitude, approach, and professional ethics of doctors, which has a paradoxical effect on those working within the Trust sector. Older doctors who were trained prior to the major macro pro-privatization adjustments heralded in by the SAPS and NEP of the early 1990s, and have established careers in the sector, primarily maintain a social justice approach to their practice, even within the structural constraints of the changing sector. In contrast, younger doctors, who are more vulnerable to market mechanisms, are structurally conditioned to employ a greater focus on market-led activities such as gaining administrative, managerial skills to make themselves more competitive in the employment market and to strategically place themselves in a position to traverse the hierarchical factions established by the older generation.

To articulate and contextualize the social environment of the hospitals, I described a particular day of fieldwork in Tayyib hospital in chapter 5 that revealed in detail the internal micropolitics of the hospital and the distrust, and rivalries between and within different medical factions. These hierarchical structures significantly impact on the everyday lives of people working in these institutions. I also described the characteristics of one of the "big-men" of the Mumbai tertiary healthcare sector, detailing how his military background and ethical comportment impacted on the organization and operations of the hospital. The emergence of medical tourism has also contributed to optimistic social and medical imaginaries of many healthcare workers. Many doctors consequently see themselves as active agents of change within the context of their professional contributions to shifting world perceptions of India in the world system.

MEDICAL TOURISM, ECONOMIC DEVELOPMENT, AND RIGHTS-BASED APPROACHES TO HEALTH

The medical tourism industry has emerged in the context of these wider, transformative global processes relating to the production, circulation, and distribution of market-led understandings of healthcare. In this sense, medical tourism can be understood as translocal, as the phenomenon is simultaneously territorialized in particular nations, yet highly mobile in the flow of people, knowledge, and capital. International experience over the course of the last half century has highlighted the central problems associated with market-driven healthcare models, where private market-led health systems have been beset with higher levels of inefficiency, inequity, and cost (Evans, 1997). There are established reasons for the expansion of market-based ideologies in healthcare, namely the distributional economic benefits it reaps for both healthcare service providers and the elite.

Medical tourism is framed as a rational economic development strategy or export niche for developing nations. However, left behind in the wake of these elite hospitals are local populations facing critical health issues, and increasing social, cultural, and economic disparities. These factors are exacerbated in many of the countries actively promoting medical tourism, in the context of incremental reduction to public health funding, while continuing in patterns of healthcare system hypercommodification. It is well recognized that these gaps are widening, yet both public and private stakeholders continue to focus resources on the development of high-cost, technologically advanced biomedical care within luxurious settings for the comparatively rich.

Here it is befitting to ask the question, will the "world class" technocratic quality improvements underway in the elite private hospitals in developing contexts such as India translate to long-term changes that will eventually permeate the entire healthcare sector? If so, at what cost? As Stiglitz (2008, 87) aptly noted, "One should not just build a bigger hospital to address public health problems." Sen (2001) too has argued that the "principal means" of development are often devalued in favor of the "primary end"; seeking the promised economic rewards (e.g. influx of foreign capital from medical tourists), while ignoring the potentially damaging outcomes that eventuate in the process of doing so.

Does India really intend on prioritizing the needs of international patients via national strategies promoting and resourcing the medical tourism trade, whilst their national population has so little access to care in the context of the hugely under resourced and ill-performing public health system? As aptly noted by Dr Rao:

> [The] disadvantage is that you are probably taking away necessary healthcare facilities from the residents of the country. It is another outsourcing of required services. We already have outsourcing of nurses, outsourcing of doctors, and now we have medical services being outsourced themselves.

There have been further claims that medical tourism will assist developing nations in the retention of in-country health personnel, stemming what is commonly referred to as the "brain drain." Although it has been suggested that there has been decreased mobility of some health professionals, there remains a vast procession of doctors and nurses that continue to flow out of the country. This is particularly striking when addressing the stark reality that the number of trained doctors outside of India is far greater than those practicing within. It also fails to consider the double-movement of healthcare professionals within the nation, from the public to the private sector, which is accelerated by medical tourism (see chapter 5). This is most concerning given associated changes within the private charitable sector, with quasi-corporatizing hospitals shifting away from social justice models toward a market-based ethos. The major dilemma posed by the dominant market-led model is related to how healthcare is distributed across a population. In the case of Mumbai, as outlined in this book, healthcare is increasingly following the law of inverse care, in that it is apportioned on the basis of wealth rather than that of need.

LOCAL BIOSOCIAL INEQUITY AND THE BIOPOLITICS OF MEDICAL TOURISM IN INDIA

Another central theme explored across the book is that of the local social and biosocial equity impacts of medical tourism, namely the structural violence it inflicts on the host population. Chapter 6 described some of the conspicuous patterns of spatial exclusion and marginalization emerging across the city of Mumbai, from gated shopping centers to the zoning of entire suburbs, of which the elite hospitals offering medical tourism are very much established. The last section of chapter 6 drew on examples from my fieldwork focusing the local biosocial context of the residents of the city, particularly their access to healthcare and understandings of health, drawing on Amartya Sen's theory of development as freedom.

This book contributes to understandings of the associations between medical tourism, the commodification and hypercommodification of healthcare, and growing healthcare inequities for the local population. By drawing on theory from critical medical anthropology and rights-based approaches, the book has assembled and analyzed a variety of data to better understand the role of medical tourism in recent shifts within the tertiary healthcare system in India. These include the alignment of hospitals to the global medical tourism supply chain and the market pressures on charitable hospitals leading to the quasi-corporate transitioning of not-for-profit hospitals. The book also adds to theoretical understandings of the varied impacts of these changes to the healthcare workforce in the context of this transitioning environment.

A central argument of this book is that the main claims directing key policy decisions about medical tourism in India rely on its potential for economic development, serving to shift the attention away from its impact on local health equity. There is a significant disconnect between the resource intensive focus of government on medical tourism, providing health services for high-cost, high-tech private care for the comparatively wealthy, and the extreme inequity experienced by the majority of the populace in the context of the overburdened, fractured public system, and transitioning charitable sector. This book has developed a conceptual framing that enables the in-depth analysis of the impact of medical tourism on the local institutions, the healthcare workforce, and the wider local population.

CHALLENGING THE NEOLIBERAL RHETORIC OF MEDICAL TOURISM

A series of neoliberal metanarratives promoting the advantages of medical tourism for the nation have been discursively constituted nationally and globally and are reproduced in the local advertising and marketing campaigns of local hospitals seeking international patient patronage. A key claim that has been locally reconstituted is that medical tourism relieves the burden of patients unable to access healthcare service in their own nations. It is this contention that raises significant questions of neo-colonialism, particularly with reference to the medical tourists originating from developed nations accessing services in developing nations. The demand for tertiary healthcare services for the Indian population is growing exponentially; yet, the spatial and cost-related barriers to accessing treatment are rapidly worsening. Alongside domestic and global market pressures, medical tourism is contributing directly and indirectly to increases in healthcare costs, with the greatest burden falling on those least able to pay. Moreover, as the benefits of the industry are structured to increase the wealth of the elite and impact detrimentally on the poor, it reinforces and polarizes the significant, deep-seated equity gaps already present.

The commodification of healthcare services within national healthcare systems have long been linked to cycles of inequality within populations globally. Examples include the increase in healthcare costs that place unsustainable financial burdens on households, causing further exclusion from care and reduction of income due to poor health and the fostering of divisive delivery of healthcare services in terms of quality, reinforcing social segregation while increasing health disparities within populations (Mackintosh 2006). Further, there is general consensus within the international community that governments should fund at least an essential or basic level of healthcare for the populace due to the failure of the market to accommodate for the negative impact it has on the resource poor (Diaz-Bonilla et al. 2002; Gupta and Dasgupta 2002; Lall and Lundberg 2006). These factors establish a theoretical case to view healthcare services as a fictional commodity. If healthcare services are indeed a fictional commodity, the hypercommodification encouraged by medical tourism can only reinforce and increase disadvantage for vulnerable groups in destination countries.

Regardless, economic development rhetoric continues to form the dominant discourse within media, government, and private sectors alike, maintaining that medical tourism will improve the Indian healthcare system and health status of the population. The general assertion made is that economic growth derived from medical tourism will be syphoned back into hospitals, improving the technology, equipment, and increase employment opportunities, benefiting the population at large. However, this argument fails to address which hospitals across the tertiary sector that will benefit from medical tourism. As discussed throughout this book, the institutions that are able to attract medical tourists are the elite, private, and (quasi)corporatized hospitals. These hospitals are generally inaccessible to the majority of the local population, and local regulations attempting to make these hospitals more inclusive are rarely enforced.

Government promotion, concessions, and incentives directed toward the medical tourism industry must be challenged in contexts where public health expenditure is consistently reduced. Although medical tourism comprises only one of many neoliberal imprints emerging in the wake of rapid global healthcare commodification, the cost of further expansion of the industry without greater consideration of how to attenuate its damage to local populations will be disastrous for the population health outcomes of India and global health en masse.

MULTI-SITED HOSPITAL ETHNOGRAPHY

This book has drawn on an array of methodological approaches, with a reliance on multi-sited ethnography—and in this case the multiple sites were (predominantly) the hospitals of the study. Accordingly, I have drawn on an array of rich observational data and interviews alongside a range of other empirical development data, such as media, government and institutional material interwoven across the chapters. One of the most significant methodological challenges when designing the research for this ethnography was determining an appropriate field for the study and the work required to understand the associations between such diverse, multi-scalar social actors and institutions. Hence, this book contributes to new ways of thinking about how to understand and study emerging social phenomena in a globalizing world. The book makes further methodological contributions to the area of hospital ethnography, particularly in the application of a multi-sited framework. Many contemporary hospital ethnographies have asserted that hospitals are a site that "both reflect and reinforce dominant social and cultural processes of their societies" (Van Der Geest and Finkler 2004, 1996). Shifting the focus of the research between different hospital sites and social and cultural locations in which the phenomenon of interest is located can both broaden and enable more nuanced understandings of particular health-related phenomena across different, yet related sites.

A key factor motivating this research was to look more closely at the local perspective of healthcare providers of medical tourism in a developing country setting in order to better understand the association to health inequities. As noted by Biehl and Petryna (2013, 3):

> By looking closely at life stories and at the ups and downs of individuals and communities as they grapple with inequality, struggle to access technology, and confront novel state-market formations, we begin to apprehend larger systems. We are able to see them in the making or in the process of dissolution, and we understand more intimately the local realities, so often unspoken, that result when people are seen or governed in a particular way, or not at all.

A practical contribution of this book is the description and analysis of some of the more significant changes occurring in the tertiary healthcare sector in India by detailing the everyday functioning in five private hospitals in Mumbai. By interrogating the interrelationships of medical tourism with processes of hypercommodification, this book has outlined specific areas in which the Indian government, and other developing nations undergoing similar transitions, can address the regulatory and policy framework to negate or lessen the impact for the most vulnerable populations.

As outlined in chapter 6, Mumbai's private hospitals are rapidly developing into differentiated islands of privilege, where the rich can quickly access high-quality services, while most of the population are facing increased barriers to access, lower quality services and higher associated costs. These findings are directly relevant and can inform government policy makers in India and other countries facing similar experiences, international institutions, the local hospitals engaging in medical tourism and even potential medical tourists to inform their decision-making processes.

The book further contributes toward a more in-depth, locally contextualized understandings of the global emergence of modern modes of medical tourism, particularly in terms of recent historical, economic, and bio-political contexts. Within the book I describe some of the broader global issues, risks, ethical concerns, and responsibilities related to the different actors engaging in medical tourism, including the industry sustaining and promoting these practices, national and local governments of incoming and outgoing medical tourists, international institutions such as the WTO, IMF, WHO and the World Bank, and the healthcare workforce.

MEDICAL TOURISM AND THE DISTORTION OF HEALTH PRIORITIES

Medical tourism has grown rapidly internationally, yet remains a distinctly understudied area. This book highlights the urgent need for richer, in-depth, and contextualized understandings of medical tourism that move beyond the prevailing, one-dimensional, market-led theoretical propositions driving the industry. The medical tourism industry in Mumbai exposes vulnerable and disadvantaged groups to further entrenchment of inequity by distorting needs-based healthcare distribution.

I do not claim that the same patterns of hypercommodification and consequent pressures of medical tourism on local equity are experienced in the same way in other contexts. However, the likelihood of similar patterns emerging in other developing host nations illustrate the urgent need for further studies of medical tourism focusing on specific contextual associations between the historical, bioethical, economic, social and political dimensions for different localities. Without further international exploration of the material impact and local manifestations of medical tourism, it is impracticable to ascertain and negotiate the value or potential pitfalls of pursuing such an industry.

Further, greater attention is required focusing on the main groups and actors that are the beneficiaries of the policies supporting medical tourism, and their role in the emergence and reformulation of the institutions the industry supports. Importantly, the major social risks created by the growth of the medical tourism industry need to be articulated in their contextual variations to enable strategies to mitigate the devastating outcomes for large sectors of the global population.

The findings set out in this book illustrate that in the race to attract greater flows of medical tourism, elite hospitals may improve their quality and standard of care provided, but by doing so, they drive increasing costs of healthcare across the entire healthcare system. Further, as competition increases in the tertiary healthcare market, hospitals that have previously provided care for the large and diverse subaltern population are less inclined to do so, leaving them at the mercy of the crumbling public healthcare system, or without any care at all.

Medical tourism influences the incorporation of expensive, lavish features provided by luxury hotels within hospitals. This was noted by Dr Lulla, "if I did not have central air conditioning, a nice ambience and such a lavish space, my capital costs would have reduced. I would have provided my services much cheaper, which means more people would have afforded it. But, yes, my medical tourist patient would not come." This is one of the factors where medical tourism has both supported and contributed to a neoliberal shift in the operational functioning of private not-for-profit hospitals. Not-for-profit hospitals that have not adapted to increase their competitiveness with the influx of corporate hospitals in Mumbai have found it extremely challenging to maintain economic viability. Those that are transitioning as a response to the changing economic conditions have shifted their varied philanthropic and religious ethos of caring for the most vulnerable, to a market-led, corporatized approach. Again, those that have moved to a market-led approach are extremely invested in improving their standards of care. Yet, the hospitals that have cared for the most vulnerable populations in the past are either disappearing or becoming less able, or less inclined, to do so.

Given the rapidly increasing population of the city and growing demand for hospital services, these structural conditions are potentially disastrous for a population of already over 21 million, nearly half of whom live in slum-like conditions. The experience of inaccessibility to healthcare services and lifesaving treatment for the local population has been highlighted by the Covid-19 pandemic, with the hoarding of medical supplies, mass migration out of urban centers, and commercialization of vaccines. The context is further compounded by the political apathy related to any moves to restructure or invest in public hospitals, which are already insufficient in number, quality and lack of resources in beds, staffing and expertise. To place this in the wider context of India's public healthcare system, Sen and Dreze (1999, 101) noted: "In some states, this system is little more than a collection of deserted primary health centers, filthy dispensaries, unmotivated doctors, and chaotic hospitals."

If medical tourism rebounds from the Covid-19 pandemic, it could bring with it a slew of advantages, disadvantages and, in some cases, little change at all for the population at large. However, what can be drawn from this book is that those who will carry the heaviest burden of the changes brought about by the phenomena are the most disadvantaged within the population. Inversely, those receiving the greatest benefit will be the elite of the nation. Even with regulatory measures in place aimed at reducing this burden—such as the policies requiring charitable hospitals to reserve one-fifth of their beds for low socioeconomic groups—the lack of compliance and enforcement exemplifies the general disinterest of those in power to shift the status quo. As noted by Sen and Dreze (1999, 93), "the positive role of the government in expanding social opportunities can be severely undermined by political pressure from privileged groups geared to the protection of sectional interests." The power of private lobby groups, including major business conglomerates and multi-national corporations, pursuing the enormous commercial profit from the tertiary healthcare industry—including medical tourism—is invisibilized by the under-politicization and failure to adequately problematize the structural power-based issues.

Medical tourism as an industry has grown exponentially in the international arena, mobilizing significant attention, but it remains a distinctly understudied area. There remains a great need for further critical scholarship examining the associations and connections between the multi-layered institutions, and social actors directing the industry with a focus on issues of inequity. In the current global economic climate, many concerning issues related to the impact of medical tourism raised in this book are only intensifying in their relevance, but remain unquestioned in mainstream, political, and scholarly parlance. In particular, the emergence of coronavirus pandemic has shone a spotlight on the extreme deficiencies of India's public health system and the problems related to a health system so heavily reliant on private health. Neoliberal policies, directly stemming from the SAPs of the early 1990s pushed pro-privatization agendas within the healthcare system, alongside benevolent rhetoric of efficiency. However, the aims of efficiency within a neoliberal framework rarely coincide with that of social justice, and more specifically, health equity. These principles have instead had the opposite effect, ensuring greater inequity in the distribution of health services, particularly in terms of access.

There is little evidence to support suggestions that market mechanisms will ensure the medical tourism industry will act as a positive force for healthcare systems in poorer countries. To the contrary, as outlined in this book, there is strong international evidence suggesting that healthcare is an area with a strong case for providing social safety nets to protect disadvantaged groups from its likely negative effects. Further, given the poor equity outcomes of past privatization reforms that have driven the hypercommodification of healthcare, it is far more likely to reinforce and widen inequity. Further, the trends emerging in Mumbai's tertiary healthcare sector suggest that it will lead to immediate, cross-sectoral price hikes, which are most damaging to the poor.

Although I have followed the tracks of the medical tourism "elephant" across temporal, multi-scalar processes and terrain, the paths traversed by this particular elephant are both highly contextualized and heterogeneous. As such, no single book can encapsulate the spectrum of the intricate interactions and dynamics occurring across variable social, cultural, economic, political, and geographic scales. However, the groups and actors who benefit most from the policies and institutions created for the promotion of medical tourism are dictated by systemic structures, and reinterpreted in local contexts, with the rules developed and set by those with the most power, and unstated vested interests. This tells us a story that we should already know. The hypercommodifying processes enabling medical tourism, where medicine and health services are treated like any other commodity to be bought and sold on the international market, present and exacerbate major social risks that are reinforced and replicated through its growth.

Glossary of Hindi Terms

Hindi	English translation
Achha	Good or okay
Auto-wallah	An auto-rickshaw driver. Auto-rickshaws are three-wheeled automobiles with no doors
Chai	Tea
Chalo	Hello, goodbye, or hurry (Strictly speaking it means "Let's Go")
Chappals	Sandals/shoes
Chawl	Low-cost rental apartments established in Mumbai in the 1920s–1950s
Churidar	Slim line pants worn under a tunic/dress (*kurta*)
Dhabba	Lunch box (A "dhaba" is a roadside eatery. The lunchbox is "dabba" without the aspirated "D")
Dhotar	The long (usually white) sheet of cloth worn by men as a lower garment, draped in a manner that outwardly looks like pants
Dupatta	Traditional Indian scarf that is draped across the front of chest
Garam	Hot
Han	Yes
Jhopadpatti	Slum (makeshift dwelling)
Kachcha	Temporary or unfixed (It means "crude." Also, can mean "raw")
Kurta	Traditional Indian tunic/dress worn over pants (churidar or salwaar)
Masjid	Mosque
Mumbaikar	A resident of Mumbai
Pani	Water
Pukka	Established/permanent (proper)
Salwaar	Baggy pants worn under a tunic/dress (kurta)
Wallah	Used as a suffix, signifying a person's occupation (e.g., a chai-wallah is a person who sells tea)

LIST OF ACRONYMS

ABPST	Adamji Peerbhoy Sanatorium Trust
AIIMS	All India Institute of Medical Sciences
AYUSH	Ayurveda, Yoga and Naturopathy, Unani, Siddha and Homeopathy
BJP	Bharatiya Janata Party
BPT	Bombay Public Trust Act, 1950
BRICS	Brazil, Russia, India, China and South Africa
CBHI	Central Bureau of Health Intelligence
CEHAT	Centre for Enquiry into Health and Allied Themes
CIE	Cambridge International Examinations
CII	Confederation of Indian Industry
ENT	Ear, Nose and Throat
ESIS	Employees State Insurance Scheme
EWS	Economically Weaker Section
FDA	Food and Drug Administration
FDI	Foreign Direct Investment
FICCI	Federation of Indian Chambers of Commerce and Industry
FICCI-MTCM	Federation of Indian Chambers of Commerce and Industry – Medical Tourism Council of Maharashtra
FIFO	Fly-in, fly-out
FYP	Five Year Plan
GATS	General Agreement on Trade and Services
GDP	Gross Domestic Product
GFC	Global Financial Crisis
ISO	International Organisation for Standardization
IITTM	Indian Institute of Tourism and Travel Management
IMF	International Monetary Fund
IMR	Infant Mortality Rate
INR	Indian National Rupee
IPF	Indigent Patients Fund
ISQua	International Society for Quality Healthcare
JCAHO	Joint Commission Accreditation, Health Care, Certification
JCI	Joint Commission International
MBBS	Bachelor of Medicine and Bachelor of Science
MHFW	Ministry of Health and Family Welfare
MOU	Memorandum of Understanding
MTC	Medical Tourism Company
NABH	National Accreditation Board for Hospitals and Health care Providers
NCD	Non-communicable disease
NDM-1	New Delhi Metallo-beta-lactamase-1
NEP	New Economic Policy
NHP	National Health Programmes
NRI	Non-Resident Indian
OECD	Organisation for Economic Cooperation and Development
PHC	Primary Health Care
POI	Person of Indian Origin
P-P-P	Private Public Partnership
PPP	Purchasing Power Parity

QCI	Quality Council of India
RIL	Reliance Industries Ltd
RLS	Reliance Life Sciences
SAL	Structural Adjustment Loan
SAP	Structural Adjustment Program
SC/ST	Scheduled Caste or Tribe
SHC	Secondary Health Care
THC	Tertiary Health Care
TISS	Tata Institute of Social Sciences
TRIPS	Trade-Related Aspects of Intellectual Property Rights
WHO	World Health Organization
WTO	World Trade Organization
UN	United Nations
UNDP	United Nations Development Program
UNESCO	United Nations Educational, Scientific and Cultural Organisation

Bibliography

Altbach, Philip G. 2014. "Why do Indians want to study abroad?" *The Hindu*, 4 September. Accessed 31 March 2015. http://www.thehindu.com/opinion/op-ed/why-do-indians-.

Adams, J. 2004. "The imagination and social life." *Qualitative Sociology* 27 (3): 277–97.

Adiga, Aravind. 2008. *The White Tiger*. Uttar Pradesh, India: Harper Collins.

Agarwal, S. 2006. "India's emerging economy: Performance and prospects in 1990s and beyond." *Finance India* 20 (2): 649–52.

Agarwal, Sanjay, and Noshir Dadrawala. 2004. "The legal context for philanthropy and law in India." In *Philanthropy and Law in South Asia*, edited by Mark Sidel and Iftekhar Zaman, 115–18. Asia Pacific Philanthropy Corsortium.

Ahasan, Rabiul, Timo Partanen, and Lee Keyoung. 2001. "Global Corporate Policy for Financing Health Services in the Third World: The Structural Adjustment Crisis." *International Quarterly of Community Health Education* 20 (1): 3–15.

Allen-Scott, L. K., J. M. Hatfield, and L. McIntyre. 2014. "A scoping review of unintended harm associated with public health interventions: Towards a typology and an understanding of underlying factors." *International Journal of Public Health* 59 (1): 3–14.

Alvaredo, Facundo, Tony Atkinson, Thomas Picketty, Emmanuel Saez, and Gabriel Zucman. 2016. "The world wealth and income database." Accessed 22 March 2016. http://www.wid.world/.

Amit, Sengupta, and Nundy Samiran. 2005. "The private health sector in India." *British Medical Journal* 331 (7526): 1157.

Anand, AC. 2003. "New managers for medical research: Superspecialists or middlemen?" *The National Medical Journal of India* 16 (4): 216–18.

Anand, Sudhir, and Amartya Sen. 2000. "Human development and economic sustainability." *World Development* 28 (12): 2029–49.

Andrews, Wilson. 2012. "The high cost of medical procedures in the U.S." *The Washington Post*. Accessed 1 March 2013. http://www.washingtonpost.com/wp-srv/special/business/high-cost-of-medical-procedures-in-the-us/.

Appadurai, Arjun, ed. 1988. *The Social Life of Things: Commodities in Cultural Perspective*. Cambridge, UK: Cambridge University Press.

Appadurai, Arjun. 1994. "Commodities and the politics of value." In *Interpreting Objects and Collections*, edited by Susan M. Pearce, 76–91. London: Routledge.

Appadurai, Arjun. 1996. *Modernity at Large: Cultural Dimensions of Globalization*. Vol. 1. Minneapolis, MN: University of Minnesota Press.

Appadurai, Arjun. 2000. "Spectral housing and urban cleansing: notes on millennial Mumbai." *Public Culture* 12 (3): 627–51.

Arnold, David. The Tropics and the Traveling Gaze: India, Landscape and Science, 1800–1856. University of Washington Press, 2006.

Arnold, David. 1993. Colonizing the Body: State Medicine and Epidemic Disease in Nineteenth-century India. Berkeley: University of California Press.

Arputham, J., and S. Patel. 2010. "Recent developments in plans for Dharavi and for the airport slums in Mumbai." *Environment and Urbanization* 22 (2): 501.

Australian Bureau of Statistics. 2012. Australian Social Trends, Dec 2011: International Students. Canberra: ABS.

Australian Institute of Health and Welfare. 2014. Australian hospital statistics 2012–13. In *Health Services Series No. 54. Cat. No. HSE 145*. Canberra: AIHW.

Baer, Hans, Merrill Singer, and Ida Susser. 2013. *Medical Anthropology and the World System: Critical Perspectives*. Third Edition. Santa Barbara, CA: Praeger.

Bajaj, A. 2021. "Healthcare industry in India is projected to research $372 bn by 2022." *Snapshot Invest India*. New Delhi: National Investment Promotion and Faciliation Agency. Accessed 29 October 2021. https://www.investindia.gov.in/sector/healthcare.

Banerji, Debabar. 1981. "The place of indigenous and western systems of medicine in the health services of India." *Social Science & Medicine. Part A: Medical Psychology & Medical Sociology* 15 (2): 109–14.

Banerji, Debabar. 1984. "The political economy of western medicine in third world countries." In *Issues in the Political Economy of Health Care*, edited by John B. McKinlay, 257–82. New York: Tavistock.

Bapat, Meera, and Indu Agarwal. 2003. "Our needs, our priorities: Women and men from the slums in Mumbai and Pune talk about their needs for water and sanitation." *Environment and Urbanization* 15 (2): 71–86. doi:10.1177/095624780301500221.

Barraclough, Simon. 1997. "Malaysia: Policy contradictions in health system pluralism." *International Journal of Health Services* 27 (4): 643, 659.

Barrett, Ron. 2008. *Aghor Medicine: Pollution, Death, and Healing in Northern India*. Oakland: University of California Press.

Baru, Rama. 2001. "Health sector reforms and structural adjustment: A state-level analysis." In *Public Health and the Poverty of Reforms: The South Asian Predicament*, edited by Imrana Qadeer, Kasturi Sen and K. R. Nayar, 211–34. New Delhi, Thousand Oaks and London: Sage Publications.

Basole, Amit. 2014. "Dynamics of income inequality in India: Insights from world top incomes database." *Economic & Political Weekly* 49 (40): 14–17.

Bennett, Jennifer. 2001. "Structural adjustment and the poor in Pakistan." In *Public Health and the Poverty of Reforms: The South Asian Predicament*, edited by Imrana Qadeer, Katsuri Sen and K. R. Nayar, 51–62. New Delhi, Thousand Oaks and London: Sage Publications.

Bhagat, R. B., and S. Mohanty. 2009. "Emerging pattern of urbanization and the contribution of migration in urban growth in India." *Asian Population Studies* 5 (1): 5–20.

Bhandari, Neena. 2015. "Is ayurveda the key to universal healthcare in India?" *BMJ* 350: 1–3. Accessed 28 May 2015. doi:10.1136/bmj.h2879.

Bhat, Ramesh. 1999. "Characteristics of private medical practice in India: A provider perspective." *Health Policy and Planning* 14 (1): 26.

Bhattacharya, Nandini. 2013. "Leisure, economy and colonial urbanism: Darjeeling, 1835–1930." *Urban History* 40 (3): 442–61.

Bhore, Joseph. 1946. Report of the Health Survey and Development Committee. edited by Health Survey and Development Committee. Calcutta (Kolkata): Government of India Press.

Bianchi, Raoul. 2009. "The 'Critical Turn' in Tourism Studies: A Radical Critique." *Tourism geographies* 11 (4): 484–504.

Biehl, João, and Adriana Petryna. 2013. *When People Come First: Critical Studies in Global Health*. Princeton University Press.

Bochaton, Audrey, and Bertrand Lefebvre. 2009. "The rebirth of the hospital: Heterotopia and medical tourism in Asia." In *Asia On Tour*, edited by Tim Winter, Peggy Teo and T. C. Chang, 97–108. New York: Routledge.

Bookman, Milica Z., and Karla R. Bookman. 2007. *Medical Tourism in Developing Countries*. New York: Palgrave Macmillan.

Bose, S. 2012. "A contextual analysis of gender disparity in education in India: The relative effects of son preference, women's status, and community." *Sociological Perspectives* 55 (1): 67–91.

Buncombe, Andrew. 2012. "The verminators: On the frontline of Mumbai's battle with 88 million rats." *The Independent*, World. Accessed 21 March 2015. http://www.independent.co.uk/news/world/asia/the-verminators-on-the-frontline-of-mumbais-battle-with-88-million-rats-8061492.html.

Caldeira, T. P. R. 2000. *City of Walls: Crime, Segregation and Citizenship in Sao Paolo*. Berkeley: University of California Press.

Canniford, R., K. Riach and T. Hill. 2018. "Nosenography: How smell constitutes meaning, identity and temporal experience in spatial assemblages." *Marketing Theory* 18 (2): 234–48.

Caton, K., H. Mair, M. Muldoon, and B. Grimwood. 2018. "Introduction: Engaging the nexus of wellness and (critical) tourism studies." In *Tourism and Wellness: Travel for the Good of All?*, edited by Bryan Grimwood, S. R. Bryan, Heather Mair, Kellee Caton, and Megan Muldoon, xv–xix. Lanham: Lexington Books.

Central Bureau of Health Intelligence. 2010. *National Health Profile 2009: 5th Issue*, edited by Ministry of Health & Family Welfare Directorate General of Health Services. New Delhi: Government of India.

Chacko, Pheba. 2005. "Medical tourism in India: Issues and challenges." ICFAI University Press.

Chakravarthi, Indira. 2011. "Corporate presence in healthcare sector in India." *Social Medicine* 5 (4): 192–204.

Chambers, E. 1997. *Tourism and Culture: An Applied Perspective*. New York: SUNY Press.

Chambers, D., and B. McIntosh. 2008. "Using authenticity to achieve competitive advantage in medical tourism in the English speaking Caribbean." *Third World Quarterly* 29: 919–37.

Chanda, Rupa. 2002. "Trade in health services." *Bulletin of the World Health Organization* 80 (2): 158–63.

Chaplin, Susan E. 1999. "Cities, sewers and poverty: India's politics of sanitation." *Environment and Urbanization* 11 (1): 145–58.

Charity Commissioner of Maharashtra. n.d. Statistics: Statement showing Information Regarding Total No. of Operational Beds and Reserved Beds by the Respective Charitable Hospitals, edited by Office of the Charity Commissioner. Pune: NIC.

Cobaj, Lee. 2014. "Thailand: What martial law has meant for tourists." *Travel*. Accessed 20 November 2015. http://www.telegraph.co.uk/travel/destinations/asia/thailand/11090003/Thailand-what-martial-law-has-meant-for-tourists.html.

Cohen, G. 2010. "Medical tourism: The view from ten thousand feet." *Hastings Center Report* 40: 11–12.

Connell, John. 2011. *Medical Tourism*. Oxfordshire, UK: CABI.

Connell, John. 2013. "Contemporary medical tourism: Conceptualisation, culture and commodification." *Tourism Management* 34: 1–13.

Connell, John. 2015. "Transnational health care: Global markets and local marginalisation in medical tourism?" In *Bodies Across Borders: The Global Circulation of Body Parts, Medical Tourists and Professionals*, edited by Bronwyn Parry, Beth Greenhough, Tim Brown and Isabel Dyck. Farnham, UK: Ashgate.

Connell, John. 2016. "Reducing the scale? From global images to border crossings in medical tourism." *Global Networks* 16 (4): 531–50.

Crooks, V. A., P. Kingsbury, J. Snyder, and R. Johnston. 2010. "What is known about the patient's experience of medical tourism? A scoping review." *BMC Health Services Research* 10: 266–78.

Dandekar, Vikas. 2016. "Reliance life sciences get US FDA nod for Navi Mumbai plant." *The Economic Times*, n.p., Healthcare. Accessed 19 February 2016. http://economictimes.indiatimes.com/industry/healthcare/biotech/healthcare/reliance-life-sciences-gets-us-fda-nod-for-navi-mumbai-plant/articleshow/50525450.cms.

Das Gupta, Monica, and Manju Rani. 2004. "India's public health system: How well does it function at the national level." In *World Bank Policy Research Working Paper 3447*. World Bank.

Das, Jishnu, and Jeffrey Hammer. 2005. "Money for nothing: The dire straits of medical practice in Delhi, India." In *World Bank Policy Research Working Paper 3669*. World Bank.

Das, Jishnu, Alaka Holla, Veena Das, Manoj Mohanan, Diana Tabak, and Brian Chan. 2012. "In urban and rural India, a standardized patient study showed low levels of provider training and huge quality gaps." *Health Affairs* 31 (12): 2774–84.

de Arellano, A. B. R. 2007. "Patients without borders: The emergence of medical tourism." *The International Journal of Health Services* 37 (1): 193–98.

de Arellano, A. B. R. 2014. "Medical tourism in the Caribbean." *Signs* 40 (1): 289–97.

de Kadt, E. 1979. "Social planning for tourism in the developing countries." *Annals of Tourism Research* 6: 36–48.

Del Vecchio Good, Mary-Jo. 1995. "Cultural studies of biomedicine: An agenda for research." *Social Science & Medicine* 41 (4): 461–73.

Del Vecchio Good, Mary-Jo. 2010. "The medical imaginary and the biotechnical embrace: Subjective experiences of clinical scientists and patients." In *A Reader in Medical Anthropology: Theoretical Trajectories, Emergent Realities*, edited by Byron J. Good, M. J. Fischer, Sarah S. Willen and Mary-Jo DelVecchio Good, 272–83. West Sussex, UK: Blackwell Publishing.

Delhi Tourism and Transport Development Corporation. 2008. "Wellness/Fitness: Medical Destinations." Accessed 3 July 2009. http://www.ibef.org/download/Health-Tourism_091211.pdf.

Denoon, David B. H. 1998. "Cycles in Indian economic liberalization 1966–1996." *Comparative Politics* 31 (1): 43–60.

Department of Industrial Policy & Promotion. 2014. *Fact Sheet on Foreign Direct Investment (FDI): From April 2000 to October 2014*, edited by Government of India. New Delhi: DIPP.

Desai, A. R. 1987. "Rural development and human rights in independent India." *Economic and Political Weekly* 22 (31): 1291–96.

Deshmukh, M. S. 2013. "Conditions of slum population of major sub-urban wards of Mumbai in Maharashtra." *Voice of Research* 2: 34–40.

Diaz-Bonilla, Eugenio, Julie Babinard, and P. Pinstrup-Anderson. 2002. "Globalization and health: A survey of opportunities and risks for the poor in developing countries." In *CMH Working Paper Series. Paper No. WG4:11.*

Di Giovine, Michael A. 2009. "Revitalization and counter-revitalization: Tourism, heritage, and the Lantern Festival as catalysts for regeneration in Hội An, Việt Nam." *Journal of Policy Research in Tourism, Leisure and Events* 1 (3): 208–30.

Directorate of Economics and Statistics. 2015. *Economic Survey of Maharashtra 2014–2015*. Mumbai: Planning Department, Government of Maharashtra.

Directorate-General of Health Services. 1983. *National Health Policy 1983*. New Delhi: India Ministry of Health & Family Welfare, Government of India.

Directorate-General of Health Services. 2002. *National Health Policy 2002*. India: Ministry of Health & Family Welfare.

Dreze, Jean, and Amartya Sen. 2002. *India: Development and Participation*. New York: Oxford University Press.

Duggal, Ravi. 2007. "Healthcare in India: Changing the financing strategy." *Social Policy and Administration* 41 (4): 386.

Duggal, Ravi. 2012. "The uncharitable trust hospitals." *Economic & Political Weekly* 47 (25): 23.

Duttagupta, Ishani. 2011. "Indian healthcare: Stop the brain drain of doctors." *The Economic Times*, Industry. Accessed 3 March 2016. http://articles.economic-times.indiatimes.com/2011-08-20/news/29909305_1_indian-doctors-physicians-of-indian-origin-british-association.

Edge, Jennifer S., and Steven J. Hoffman. 2013. "Empirical impact evaluation of the WHO global code of practice on the international recruitment of health personnel in Australia, Canada, UK and USA." *Globalization and Health* 9 (1): 60.

Eriksen, Thomas Hylland. 2014. *Globalization: The Key Concepts*. A&C Black.

Engineer, Asghar Ali. 1979. "The bohras: Bound by terror." *Economic and Political Weekly* 14 (23): 964–966.

Ernst & Young. 2006. *Healthcare Industry*. New Delhi: India Brand Equity Foundation (IBEF).

Escobar, Arturo. 2004. "Development, violence and the new imperial order." *Development* 47 (15): 15–21.

Evans, Catrin, Rafath Razia, and Elaine Cook. 2013. "Building nurse education capacity in India: Insights from a faculty development programme in Andhra Pradesh." *BMC Nursing* 12 (1): 1–8.

Evans, Robert G. 1997. "Going for the gold: The redistributive agenda behind market-based health care reform." *Journal of Health Politics, Policy and Law* 22 (2): 427–65.

Falzon, Mark-Anthony, ed. 2016. *Multi-sited Ethnography: Theory, Praxis and Locality in Contemporary Research*. 2nd ed. London & New York: Routledge.

Farmer, Paul. 1999. "Pathologies of power: Rethinking health and human rights." *American Journal of Public Health* 89 (10): 1486–96.

Farmer, Paul. 2005. *Pathologies of Power: Health, Human Rights, and the New War on the Poor*. 2nd ed. Berkeley: University of California Press.

Farmer, Paul, Arthur Kleinman, Jim Kim, and Matthew Basilico. 2013. *Reimagining Global Health: An Introduction*. Vol. 26. Berkeley and Los Angeles, California: University of California Press.

FDI India. 2021. "Sectors: Healthcare." New Delhi: FDI India. Accessed 11 June 2021. https://www.fdi.finance/sectors/healthcare.

Feachem, Richard G. A. 2000. "Poverty and inequity: A proper focus for the new century." *Bulletin of the World Health Organization* 78 (1): 1–2.

Featherstone, Michael. 1995. Undoing Culture: Globalisation, Postmodernism and Identity. London: Sage.

Federation of Indian Chambers of Commerce and Industry – Medical Tourism Council of Maharashta. 2003. "About FICCI-MTCM." New Delhi: Government of India. Accessed 20 September 2011. http://www.ficci-mtcm.com.

Federation of Indian Chambers of Commerce and Industry. 2020. "Travel and tourism: Survive, revive and thrive in times of COVID-19." New Delhi: Grant-Thornton India. https://www.grantthornton.in/globalassets/1.-member-firms/india/assets/pdfs/travel-and-tourism-covid-19-24-june-2020.pdf.

Fochsen, Grethe, Kirti Deshpande, and Anna Thorson. 2006. "Power imbalance and consumerism in the doctor-patient relationship: Health care providers' experiences of patient encounters in a rural district in India." *Qualitative Health Research* 16 (9): 1236–51.

Forsythe, Diana E. 1999. ""It's just a matter of common sense": Ethnography as invisible work." *Computer Supported Cooperative Work (CSCW)* 8 (1): 127–45.

Frank, Andre Gunder. 1969. *Latin America and Underdevelopment*. New York: Monthly Review Press.

Frank, Andre Gunder. 1978. *Dependent Accumulation and Underdevelopment*. London: Macmillan.

Frank, Andre Gunder. 1984. Critique and Anti-critique: Essays on Dependence and Reformism. London: Macmillan.

Friedman, Jonathan, and Kajsa Ekholm Friedman. 2013. "Globalization as a discourse of hegemonic crisis: A global systemic analysis." *American Ethnologist* 40 (2): 244–57.

Gale, Jason. 2015. "How Thailand became a global gender-change destination." *Bloomberg Business*, October 27. Accessed 23 November 2015. http://www.bloomberg.com/news/features/2015-10-26/how-thailand-became-a-global-gender-change-destination.

Gale, Tim. 2008. "The end of tourism, or endings in tourism." In *Tourism and Mobilities: Local-Global Connections*, edited by Peter M. Burns and Marina Novelli, 1–14. Oxfordshire, UK: CAB International.

Gangolli, Leena V., Ravi Duggal, and Abhay Shukla. 2005. *Review of Healthcare in India*. Mumbai: Centre for Enquiry into Health and Allied Themes Mumbai (CEHAT).

Gaventa, John. 2002. "Introduction: Exploring citizenship, participation and accountability." *IDS Bulletin* 33 (2): 1–14.

Garg, Charu C., and Anup K. Karan. 2004. "Health and millennium development goal 1: Reducing out-of-pocket expenditures to reduce income poverty – evidence from India." In *EQUITAP Project: Working Paper #15*. New Delhi: Institute for Human Development.

Ghertner, D. Asher. 2011. "Rule by aesthetics: World-class city making in Delhi." In *Worlding Cities: Asian Experiments and the Art of Being Global*, edited by Roy Ananya and Aihwa Ong, 279–306. Oxford: Wiley Blackwell.

Gisselquist, Rachel, and Anustup Kundu. 2020. *Horizontal Inequality, COVIE-19, and Lockdown Readiness: Evidence from India*. WIDER Working Paper 2020/156. Helsinki, Finland: United Nations University World Institute for Development Economics Research.

Global Association of Physicians of Indian Origin. 2016. "Introduction of GAPIO." GAPIO. Accessed 3 March 2016. http://www.gapio.in/.

Goldman, Michael. 2011. "Speculating on the Next World City." In *Worlding Cities: Asian Experiments and the Art of Being Global*, edited by Roy Ananya and Aihwa Ong, 229–58. Oxford: Wiley Blackwell.

Goodrich, Jonathan N. 1993. "Socialist Cuba: A study of health tourism." *Journal of Travel Research* 32 (1): 36–42.

Goodrich, Jonathan N., and Grace E. Goodrich. 1987. "Health-care tourism – an exploratory study." *Tourism Management* 8 (3): 217–22.

Government of India. 2001. *Census 2001 Data*. Ministry of Home Affairs and Office of the Registrar General and Census Commissioner. New Delhi: Government of India.

Government of India. 2006. "Slum data: Primary census data." In *Census of India 2001*. New Delhi: Office of the Registrar General.

Government of India. 2011. *Census 2011 data*. Ministry of Home Affairs and Office of the Registrar General and Census Commissioner. New Delhi: Government of India.

Government of India Planning Commission. 2002. "Five year plans: 1st-10th." Accessed 8 August 2005. http://planningcommission.nic.in/plans/planrel/fiveyr/default.html.

Government of India Planning Commission. 2013. *Press Note on Poverty Estimates, 2011–2012*. New Delhi: Planning Commission.

Government of India. 2020. *Sex Ratio (Females/1000 Males)*. New Delhi, India: NITI Aayog. https://niti.gov.in/content/sex-ratio-females-1000-males.

Graham, Stephen, Renu Desai, and Colin McFarlane. 2013. "Water wars in Mumbai." *Public Culture* 25 (169): 115–41.

Graburn, N. H. 2012. "The dark is on the inside: The honne of Japanese exploratory tourists." In *Emotion in Motion: Tourism, Affect and Transformation*, edited by D. Picard and M. Robinson, 49–72. London: Ashgate.

Gray, H., and S. Poland. 2008. "Medical tourism: Crossing borders to access health care." *Kennedy Institute of Ethics Journal* 18: 193–201.

Greene, Sara S. 2019. "A theory of poverty: Legal immobility." *Washington University Law Review* 96 (4): 753. Accessed 22 June 2021. https://openscholarship.wustl.edu/law_lawreview/vol96/iss4/6.

Grimwood, Bryan S. R., Heather Mair, Kellee Caton, and Meghan Muldoon, eds. 2018. *Tourism and Wellness: Travel for the Good of All?*. Lanham: Lexington Books. Accessed October 25, 2021. ProQuest Ebook Central.

Guiry, Michael. 2010. "Brand positioning in the medical tourism industry: A brand personality perspective." *International Journal of Behavioural and Healthcare Research* 2 (1): 20–37.

Gupta, Akhil. 2012. *Red Tape: Bureaucracy, Structural Violence, and Poverty in India*. Durham, North Carolina: Duke University Press.

Gupta, Akhil, and James Ferguson. 1997. *Culture, Power, Place: Explorations in Critical Anthropology*. Durham, North Carolina: Duke University Press.

Gupta, Akhil, and Aradhana Sharma. 2006. "Globalization and Postcolonial States." *Current Anthropology* 47 (2): 277–308.

Gupta, Amit Sen 2004. "Medical tourism and public health." *People's Democracy* 27 (19): 9.

Gupta, Indrani, and Purnamita Dasgupta. 2002. "Demand for curative health care in rural India: Choosing between private, public and no care." In *Working Paper Series No. 82*. University Enclave, Delhi: National Council of Applied Economic Research.

Gupta, Indrani. 2004. "Commercial Presence in the Hospital Sector under GATS: A Case Study of India." *Journal of International and Area Studies* 11 (2): 17–43. http://www.jstor.org/stable/43111447.

Gupta, Kamla, Fred Arnold, and H. Lhungdim. 2009. "Health and living conditions in eight Indian cities." In *National Family Health Survey (NFHS-3), India, 2005–06*. Calverton, Maryland and Mumbai: International Institute for Population Sciences.

Gusterson, Hugh. 1997. "Studying Up Revisited." *PoLAR: Political & Legal Anthropology Review* 20 (1): 114–19.

Halfpenny, Kate. 2019. "The strict and not-so-strict rules for airline cabin crews' grooming and make-up." *The New Daily*, March 5. Accessed 20 June 2021. https://thenewdaily.com.au/entertainment/style/2019/03/05/rules-airline-cabin -crew-grooming/.

Han, Heesup, Yunhi Kim, Chulwon Kim, and Sunny Ham. 2015. "Medical hotels in the growing healthcare business industry: Impact of international travelers' perceived outcomes." *Journal of Business Research* 68 (9): 1869–77.

Hansen, Thomas Blom. 2005. "Sovereigns beyond the state: On legality and authority in urban India." In *Sovereign Bodies: Citizens, Migrants, and States in the Postcolonial World*, edited by Thomas Blom Hansen and Finn Stepputat, 169–91. Oxfordshire, UK: Princeton University Press.

Hannam, Kevin, and Anya Diekmann. 2010. *Tourism Development in India: A Critical Introduction*. London and New York: Routledge.

Hay, Iain, and Samantha Muller. 2014. "Questioning generosity in the golden age of philanthropy: Towards critical geographies of super-philanthropy." *Progress in Human Geography* 38 (5): 635–53.

Henderson, S., and A. R. Petersen (Eds.). 2002. *Consuming Health: The Commodification of Health Care*. London: Routledge.

Henderson, Joan C. 2004. "Healthcare tourism in Southeast Asia." *Tourism Review International* 7: 111–21.

Himmelstein, David, and Steffie Woolhandler. 2008. "Privatization in a publicly funded health care system: The U.S. experience." *International Journal of Health Services* 38 (3): 407–19.

Hiranandani Hospital. 2015. "Communities that Create." Accessed 20 July 2016. http://Ramrakhyani.com/Vision_Mission.aspx.

Hoffman, Leon, Valorie A. Crooks, Jeremy Snyder, and Krystyna Adams. 2015. "Health Equity Impacts of Medical Tourism in the Caribbean: The Need to Provide Actionable Guidance Regarding Balancing Local and Foreign Interests." *WIMJ Open* 2 (3): 142–45.

Holliday, R., D. Bell, M. Jones, K. Hardy, E. Hunter, E. Probyn, and J. Taylor. 2015. "Beautiful face, beautiful place: relational geographies and gender in cosmetic surgery tourism websites." *Gender, Place and Culture* 22 (1): 90–106. doi:10.108 0/0966369X.2013.832655.

Holmes, Douglas, and George E. Marcus. 2006. "Fast capitalism: Para-ethnography and the rise of the symbolic analyst." In *Frontiers of Capital: Ethnographic Reflections on the New Economy*, edited by Melissa S. Fisher and Greg Downey, 33–57. Durham, NC: Duke University Press.

Hong, Evelyne. 2000. "Globalisation and the impact on health: A third world view." In *Imapct of SAPs in the Third World Issue Papers*. People's Health Movement. Accessed 13 September 2016. http://phmovement.org/pdf/pubs/phm-pubs-hong.pdf.

Hooda, Shailender Kumar. 2015. "Foreign investment in hospital sector in India: Trends, patterns and issues." In *ISID Working Paper 181*. New Delhi: Institute for Studies in Industrial Development.

Horton, S., and S. Cole. 2011. "Medical returns: Seeking health care in Mexico." *Social Science and Medicine* 72 (11): 1846–52.

Human Rights Office of the High Commissioner. 2016. *Access to Medicines – A Fundamental Element of the Right to Health.* Geneva: United Nations.

Illing, Kai. 2016. "Medical hotels." In *The Routledge Handbook of Health Tourism*, edited by Melanie Kay Smith and László Puczkó, 246–60. Abingdon, Oxon: Routledge.

India Brand Equity Foundation. 2021. "Indian Healthcare Industry in India.", New Delhi. IBEF, accessed 21 February 2022. https://www.ibef.org/industry/health-care-india.aspx.

India Brand Equity Foundation. 2021. *Tourism and Hospitality.* New Delhi: IBEF. Accessed 5 June 2021. https://www.ibef.org/industry/tourism-hospitality-india/infographic.

Indian Institute of Tourism and Travel Management. 2011. *A Study of Problems and Challenges Faced by Medical Tourists Visiting India*, edited by Government of India Ministry of Tourism. New Delhi.

Indian Medical Council (Professional Conduct, Etiquette and Ethics) Regulations, 2002, Rule/Reg. Part III, Section 4. India.

Inhorn, Marcia C. 2004. "Privacy, privatization, and the politics of patronage: Ethnographic challenges to penetrating the secret world of Middle Eastern, hospital-based in vitro fertilization." *Social Science & Medicine* 59 (10): 2095–108.

Inhorn, Marcia C. 2011. "Diasporic dreaming: Return reproductive tourism to the Middle East." *Reproductive Biomedicine Online* 23 (5): 582–91.

Inhorn, M. C. and P. Patrizio. 2009. "Rethinking reproductive "tourism" as reproductive "exile"." *Fertility and Sterility* 92 (3): 904–6.

International Society for Quality in Health Care. 2015. "Accedited by ISQua." ISQua Ltd. Accessed 20 November 2015. http://www.isqua.org/accreditation/accredited -by-isqua.

Jaffrelot, C. and V. Jumle. 2020. Private Healthcare in India: Boons and Banes. *Articles - 3 November.* Paris: Institut Montaigne. Accessed 29 October 2021. https://www.institutmontaigne.org/en/blog/private-healthcare-india-boons-and-banes.

Jagannathan, Srinath, and Rajnish Rai. 2021. "The necropolitics of neoliberal state response to the Covid-19 pandemic in India." *Organization.* May 2021. https://doi.org/10.1177/13505084211020195.

James, Paul. 2005. "Arguing globalizations: Propositions towards an investigation of global formation." *Globalizations* 2 (2): 193–209.

Jhala, C. I. 2012. "The Hippocratic oath: A comparative analysis of the ancient text's relevance to American and Indian modern medicine." *Indian Journal of Pathology & Microbiology* 55 (3): 279.

Jhala, Chandrakant I., and Khushboo N. Jhala. 2012. "The Hippocratic oath: A comparative analysis of the ancient text's relevance to American and Indian modern medicine." *Indian Journal of Pathology and Microbiology* 55 (3): 279.

John, Shobha. 2011. "Medical tourism in the superbug age." *Times of India*, 17 April, Deep Focus. Accessed 18 April 2013. http://timesofindia.indiatimes.com/

home/sunday-times/deep-focus/Medical-tourism-in-the-superbug-age/articleshow /8001972.cms.

Joint Commission International. 2011. "JCI accreditation and certification: JCI accredited." Accessed 8 December. http://www.jointcommissioninternational.org /JCI-Accredited-Organizations/.

Joint Commission International. 2021. "JCI accredited organizations." Oakbrooks: JCI. Accessed 15 Jun 2021. https://www.jointcommissioninternational.org/about -jci/accredited-organizations/#.

Justice, Christopher. 1997. *Dying the Good Death: The Pilgrimage to Die in India's Holy City*. Albany: State University of New York Press.

Khandelwal, B. 2011. "'Superbug' ploy to hit Indian medical tourism." *The Indian Express*. Accessed 29 October 2021. http://www.newindianexpress.com/nation/ article230269.ece?service=print.

Kangas, Beth. 2002. "The lure of technology: Yemenis' international medical travel in a global era." Doctor of Philosophy, Department of Anthropology, The University of Arizona.

Kangas, Beth. 2007. "Hope from abroad in the international medical travel of Yemeni patients." *Anthropology and Medicine* 14 (3): 293–305.

Kangas, Beth. 2010. "Traveling for medical care in a global world." *Medical Anthropology* 29 (4): 344–62.

Kansal, Nikita. 2021. "COVID-19 hitting India's poor the hardest." *Economics, Politics and Public Policy in East Asia and the Pacific*, 18 May. Accessed 20 June 2021. https://www.eastasiaforum.org/2021/05/18/covid-19-hitting-indias-poor-the -hardest/.

Karan, Anup, Himanshu Negandhi, Rajesh Nair, Anjali Sharma, Ritika Tiwari, and Sanjay Zodpey. 2019. "Size, composition and distribution of human resource for health in India: New estimates using National Sample Survey and Registry data." *BMJ Open* 9 (4): e025979.

Karmali, Naazneen. 2011. "The world's billionaires 2011: The India story." *Forbes Magazine*. Accessed 18 December 2011. http://www.forbes.com/sites/naazneenkar-mali/2011/03/10/the-worlds-billionaires-2011the-india-story/?partner=contextstory.

Karmali, Naazneen. 2021. "India's richest billionaires 2021." *Forbes Magazine*. Accessed 7 May 2021. https://www.forbes.com/sites/naazneenkarmali/2021/04/06 /indias-10-richest-billionaires-2021/?sh=4c3f657159b7.

Karn, S. Kumar, and H. Harada. 2002. "Field survey on water supply, sanitation and associated health impacts in urban poor communities - A case from Mumbai City, India." *Water Science & Technology* 46 (11): 269–75.

Kazmi, A. 2008. "A proposed framework for strategy implementation in the Indian context." *Management Decision* 46 (10): 1564–81.

Kerr, Eve A., Elizabeth A. McGlynn, John Adams, Joan Keesey, and Steven M. Asch. 2004. "Profiling the quality of care in twelve communities: Results from the CQI study." *Health Affairs* 23 (3): 247–56.

Keshavjee, MD Salmaan. 2014. *Blind Spot: How Neoliberalism Infiltrated Global Health*. Vol. 30. Berkeley and Los Angeles, California: University of California Press.

Khan, A. Q. 2001. "Health services in Bangladesh: Development and structural reforms." In *Public Health and the Poverty of Reforms*, edited by Imrana Qadeer, Kasturi Sen and K. R. Nayar, 292–310. New Delhi, Thousand Oaks & London: Sage Publications.

Kindig, D., and G. Stoddart. 2003. "What is population health?" *American Journal of Public Health* March: 380–383. https://doi.org/10.2105/AJPH.93.3.380.

Kishimoto, Marima. 2021. "Asia medical tourism catches cold from COVID travel curbs." 2021. *Nikkei Asia*, 7 May. Accessed 19 June 2021. https://asia.nikkei.com /Business/Health-Care/Asia-medical-tourism-catches-cold-from-COVID-travel -curbs.

KPMG. 2016. *Healthcare in India: Current State and Key Imperatives*. New Delhi: KPMG India. Accessed 13 June 2021. https://assets.kpmg/content/dam/kpmg/in/ pdf/2016/09/AHPI-Healthcare-India.pdf.

Koch, Erin. 2014. *Blind Spot: How Neoliberalism Infiltrated Global Health*. Salmaan Keshavjee. Oakland: University of California Press, 2014, 240 pp. Wiley Online Library.

Kohn, T. K. 2010. "The role of serendipity and memory in experiencing fields." In *The Ethnographic Self as Resource: Writing Memory and Experience into Ethnography*, edited by Peter Collins and Anselma Gallinat, 185–99. New York: Berghahn Books.

Kopytoff, Igor. 1986. "The cultural biography of things: Commoditization as process." *The Social Life of Things: Commodities in Cultural Perspective* 68: 70–73.

Kumar, Pranav. 2006. South Asian Agenda for Services Negotiations: Commonalities & Differences. CUTS International.

Kumarasamy, Karthikeyan K., Mark A. Toleman, Timothy R. Walsh, Jay Bagaria, Fafhana Butt, Ravikumar Balakrishnan, Uma Chaudhary, Michel Doumith, Christian G Giske, and Seema Irfan. 2010. "Emergence of a new antibiotic resistance mechanism in India, Pakistan, and the UK: A molecular, biological, and epidemiological study." *The Lancet Infectious Diseases* 10 (9): 597–602.

Kumari, Minakshee. 2017. "From oscruity to a sub-divisional headquarter: Siliguri in colonial period." *Karatoya: NUB J. Hist.* 10: 210–31.

Kurian, Oommen C. 2013. Free Medical Care to the Poor: The Case of State Aided Charitable Hospitals in Mumbai. Mumbai: CEHAT.

Labonté, Ronald, and David Stuckler. 2015. "The rise of neoliberalism: How bad economics imperils health and what to do about it." *Journal of Epidemiology and Community Health*: 312–18.

Laing and Weiler. 2008. "Mind, Body and Spirit: Health and Wellness Tourism in Asia." In *Asian Tourism: Growth and Change*, edited by Janet Cochrane, 379–90. Oxford: Elsevier.

Lall, Somik V., and Mattias Lundberg. 2006. "What are public services worth, and to whom? Non-parametric estimation of capitalization in Pune." In *World Bank Policy Research Working Paper 3924*. Washington, D.C.: World Bank.

Latouche, Serge. 1993. In the Wake of the Affluent Society: An Exploitation of Post-Development. London: Zed Books.

Lautier, Marc. 2008. "Export of health services from developing countries: The case of Tunisia." *Social Science & Medicine* 67 (1): 101–10.

Layak, Suman, and Geetanjali Shukla. 2012. "Changing its DNA." In *Business Today*. Noida, India: Living Media India Ltd.

Le Draoulec, Pascale. 2007. "India's 10 top luxury hotels." *Forbes Media LLC*. Last Modified 16 November. Accessed 27 June 2012. http://www.forbes.com/2007/11/16/hotels-top-india-forbeslife-cx_pl_1116hotelsindia.html.

Lechner, Frank J. 2014. *The Globalization Reader*. John Wiley & Sons.

Lee, Hwee, and Yudi Fernando. 2015. "The antecedents and outcomes of the medical tourism supply chain." *Tourism Management* 46: 148–57.

Lefebvre, Bertrand. 2009. "'Bringing world-class health care to India': The rise of corporate hospitals." In *Indian Health Landscapes under Globalization*, edited by Alain Vaguet, 83–99. New Delhi: Manohar Publishers & Distributors.

Lefebvre, Bertrand. 2010. *Hospital Chains in India: The Coming of Age?* Paris: Asie Visions 23.

Lehmann, Uta, and Lucy Gilson. 2013. "Actor interfaces and practices of power in a community health worker programme: A South African study of unintended policy outcomes." *Health Policy and Planning* 28 (4): 358–66.

Levy, Francesca. 2010. "Mukesh Ambani's skyscraper mansion is the world's most expensive home." Accessed 14 October 2015. http://www.forbes.com/sites/francescalevy/2010/10/14/mukesh-ambani-skyscraper-mansion-carlos-slim-billionaires/.

Lipsitz, Lewis A. 2012. "Understanding health care as a complex system: The foundation for unintended consequences." *JAMA* 308 (3): 243–44.

London, Leslie, and Helen Schneider. 2012. "Globalisation and health inequalities: Can a human rights paradigm create space for civil society action?" *Social Science & Medicine* 74 (1): 6–13.

Lunt, Neil, Ki Jin, Daniel Horsfall, and Johanna Hanefeld. 2014. "Insights on medical tourism: Markets as networks and the role of strong ties." *Korean Social Science Journal* 41 (1): 19–37.

McFarlane, Colin. 2012. "From sanitation inequality to malevolent urbanism: The normalisation of suffering in Mumbai." *Geoforum* 43 (6): 1287–90.

McIntyre, Di, Lucy Gilson, Haroon Wadee, Michael Thiede, and Okore Okarafor. 2006. "Commercialisation and extreme inequality in health: The policy challenges in South Africa." *Journal of International Development* 18: 435–46.

McKinlay, John B., ed. 1985. Issues in the Political Economy of Health Care, Contemporary Issues in Health, Medicine, and Social Policy. New York: Tavistock Publications.

MacCannell, Dean. 1976. *The Tourist: A New Theory of the Leisure Class*. University of California Press.

MacCannell, D. 1992. *Empty Meeting Grounds: The Tourist Papers*. London: Psychology Press.

Mackintosh, Maureen. 2006. "Commercialisation, inequality and the limits to transition in health care: A polanyian framework for policy analysis." *Journal of International Development* 18: 393–406.

Mackintosh, Maureen, and Sergey Kovalev. 2006. "Commercialisation, inequality and transition in health care: The policy challenges in developing and transitional countries." *Journal of International Development* 18: 387–91.

MacReady, Norra. 2007. "Developing countries court medical tourists." *The Lancet* 369 (9576): 1849.

Madhiwalla, Neha. 2003. "Hospitals and city health." In *Bombay and Mumbai: The City in Transition*, edited by Sujata Patel and Jim Masselos, 111–33. New Delhi: Oxford University Press.

Madhoc, Diksha. 2021. "India's billionaires got richer while coronavirus pushed millions of vulnerable people into poverty." *CNN Business*. July 6. https://edition.cnn.com /2021/07/05/economy/ambani-adani-india-covid-billionaires-intl-hnk/index.html.

Mahal, Ajay, Abdo S. Yazbek, David H. Peters, and G.N.V. Ramana. 2001. "The Poor and Health Service Use in India." In *Health, Nutrition and Population Discussion Paper*. Washington, D.C.: World Bank.

Mandhani, Apoorva. 2021. "Comfortable stay, meals, wifi – hotels are now offering 'Covid vaccination packages'." *ThePrint*. 29 May. Accessed 20 June. https:// theprint.in/india/comfortable-stay-meals-wifi-hotels-are-now-offering-covid-vac cination-packages/667773/.

Marson, Duncan. 2011. "From mass tourism to niche tourism." In *Research Themes for Tourism*, edited by Peter Robinson, Sine Heitmann and Peter Dieke, 1–16. Oxfordshire, UK: CAB International.

Marx, Karl. 1906. *Capital: A Critique of Political Economy, Vol. I. The Process of Capitalist Production*. Translated by Frederick Engels, Ernest Untermann Eds., Samuel Moore and Edward Aveling. Chicago: Charles H. Kerr and Co.

Mathur, N. 2010. "Shopping malls, credit cards and global brands: Consumer culture and lifestyle of India's new middle class." *South Asia Research* 30 (3): 211–31.

Mazzarella, William. 2003. Shoveling Smoke: Advertising and Globalization in Contemporary India. Durham, NC: Duke University Press.

Mazumdar, Sumit. 2014. "The murky waters of medical practice in India: Ethics, economics and politics of healthcare." *Economics and Politics of Healthcare* 1 (29): 40–45.

Medhekar, Anita, and Farooq Haq. 2018. "Halal branding for medical tourism: Case of Indian hospitals." In *Digital Marketing and Consumer Engagement: Concepts, Methodologies, Tools, and Applications*. edited by Management Association, Information Resources, 1190–1212. Hershey, PA: IGI Global. http:// doi:10.4018/978-1-5225-5187-4.ch061.

Mehotra, N., and A. Ghosal. 2021. "Medical students bulwark of pandemic." *Global News*. April 27. Accessed 20 June 2021. https://globalnews.ca/news/7812527/india -healthcare-covid-19-medical-students/.

Mehta, Suketu. 2004. *Maximum City: Bombay Lost and Found*. New York: Vintage Books.

Menon, Shruti. 2021. "India coronavirus: What is the government's change to vaccine policy?" *BBC News*. 9 June. Accessed 20 June 2021. https://www.bbc.com/ news/57400891.

Merino, D., and G. Ware. 2021. "India: Why it's so hard to get a coronavirus vaccine." *The Conversation Weekly Podcast*. May 19. Accessed 20 June 2021. https:// theconversation.com/india-why-its-so-hard-to-get-a-coronavirus-vaccine-160876.

Mies, Maria, and Vandana Shiva. 1993. *Ecofeminism*. London: Fernwood Publications.

Mili, D. 2011. "Migration and healthcare: Access to healthcare services by migrants settled in Shivaji Nagar Slum of Mumbai, India." *The Health* 2 (3): 82–85.

Milstein, Arnold, and Mark Smith. 2006. "America's new refugees – Seeking affordable surgery offshore." *The New England Journal of Medicine* 355 (16): 1637.

Mines, Mattison, and Vijayalakshmi Gourishankar. 1990. "Leadership and individuality in South Asia: The case of the South Indian Big-man." *The Journal of Asian Studies* 49 (4): 761.

Ministry of AYUSH. 2021. *Summary of Infrastructure Facilities under Ayush*. New Delhi: Government of India. Accessed 21 June 2021. https://main.ayush.gov.in/infrastructure/summary-of-infrastructure-facilities-under-ayush/.

Ministry of Health & Family Welfare. 2004. *Annual Report 2003–04*. New Delhi: Government of India.

Ministry of Health & Family Welfare. 2005. *Report of the National Commission on Macroeconomics and Health*. New Delhi: World Health Organization.

Ministry of Health & Family Welfare. 2006. *2005–2006 Annual Report*. New Delhi: Government of India.

Ministry of Statistics & Programme Implementation. 2013. *Statistical Year Book, India 2013*. New Delhi: Government of India.

Ministry of Tourism. 2006. *Incredible India*. New Delhi: Government of India.

Ministry of Tourism. 2019. *India: Tourism Statistics 2019*. New Delhi: Government of India.

Mishra, P. K., Himanshu B. Rout, and Smita S. Mohapatra. 2011. "Causality between tourism and economic growth: Empirical evidence from India." *European Journal of Social Sciences* 18 (4): 518–27.

Mohan, Giles, and Jeremy Holland. 2001. "Human rights & development in Africa: Moral intrusion or empowering opportunity?" *Review of African Political Economy* 28 (88): 177–96.

Mondal, Samir K., and Vineeta Kanwal. 2006. "Addressing key issues in the light of Structural Adjustment Programme (SAP) in health and family welfare sector in India." In *Working Paper*. New Delhi: National Council of Applied Economic Research (NCAER).

Morgan, L. M. 1990. "The medicalization of anthropology: A critical perspective on the critical-clinical debate." *Social Science & Medicine* 30 (9): 945–50.

Moufakkir, Omar, and Peter M. Burns, eds. 2012. *Controversies in Tourism*. Oxfordshire, UK: CAB International.

Mudur, Ganapati. 2015. "Experts question how India will meet promises on public health after cut in budget for 2015–16." *BMJ* 350: 1244.

Mukherjee, S. 2010. "Leisure and recreation in colonial Bengal: A socio-cultural study." *Proceedings of the Indian History Congress* 71: 764–73.

Mullan, Fitzhugh. 2006. "Doctors for the world: Indian physician emigration." *Health Affairs* 25 (2): 380.

Murphy, P. E. 1985. *Tourism: A Community Approach*. New York: Methuen.

Nader, Laura. 1969. "Up the anthropologics: Perspectives gained from studying up." In *Reinventing Anthropology*, edited by Dell Hymes, 1–28. New York: Random House.

National Accreditation Board for Hospitals & Healthcare Providers. 2015. "NABH Accredited Hospitals." Quality Council of India. Accessed 20 November 2015. http://nabh.co/Hospitals.aspx.

Narayan, K. N. 2011. "Turning the searchlight within, presidential address on the eve of Republic Day, 25 January 2000. In *In the Name of the People: Reflections on Democracy, Freedom and Development*, 145–49. New Delhi: Penguin Books India.

National Health Accounts Cell. 2005. *National Health Accounts India 2001–2002*. New Delhi: Ministry of Health and Family Welfare, Government of India.

National Sample Survey Organisation. 1998. "Morbidity and treatment of ailments." In *NSS Fifty-second Round July 1995-June 1996*. New Delhi: Department of Statistics, Government of India.

National Sample Survey Office. 2006. "Morbidity, health care and the condition of the aged: NSS 60th round." In *Report No. 507*. New Delhi: Ministry of Statistics and Programme Implementation, Government of India.

National Sample Survey Office. 2014. *Health in India*. New Delhi, India: Government of India. http://mospi.nic.in/sites/default/files/publication_reports/nss_rep574.pdf.

National Statistical Office. 2020. *Health in India: NSS 75th Round*. New Delhi, India: Ministry of Statistics and Programme Implementation. Government of India. Accessed 13 June 2021. http://mospi.nic.in/sites/default/files/publication_reports/NSS%20Report%20no.%20586%20Health%20in%20India.pdf.

Navarro, V. 1988. "Professional dominance or proletarianization?: Neither." *The Milbank Quarterly*: 57–75.

Naydenova E., A. Raghu, J. Ernst, S. A. Sahariah, M. Gandhi, and G. Murphy. 2018. "Healthcare choices in Mumbai slums: A cross-sectional study." *Wellcome Open Res.* 5 (2): 115.

Nazir, Zeenat. 2006. "Just what the hospital ordered: Global accreditations." *The Indian Express*, Business. http://www.indianexpress.com/story/12890.html.

Ng, Carl Jon Way. 2019. ""You are your only limit": Appropriations and valorizations of affect in university branding." *Journal of Sociolinguistics* 23 (2): 121–39.

Nussbaum, Martha C. 1997. "Capabilities and human rights." *Fordham Law Review* 66: 273.

Ong, Aihwa. 1999. Flexible Citizenship: The Cultural Logics of Transnationality. Durham, NC: Duke University Press.

Ong, A., and S. J. Collier. 2005. *Global Assemblages: Technology, Politics, and Ethics as Anthropological Problems*. Malden, MA; Oxford: Blackwell Publishing.

Ong, Aihwa, and Nancy N. Chen, eds. 2010. *Asian Biotech: Ethics and Communities of Fate*. Durham: Duke University Press.

Ong, Aihwa. 2016. *Fungible Life: Experiment in the Asian City of Life*. Durham, NC: Duke University Press.

Ormond, Meghann. 2014. "Medical tourism." In *The Wiley Blackwell Companion to Tourism*, edited by Alan A. Lew, C. Michael Hall and Allan M. Williams, 425–34. Malden, MA: John Wiley & Sons.

Ormond, Meghann. 2015. "Solidarity by demand? Exit and voice in international medical travel – The case of Indonesia." *Social Science and Medicine* 124: 305–12.

Ormond, Meghann, and Heidi Kaspar. 2018. "South-south medical tourism." In *Routledge Handbook of South-South Relations*, edited by Elena Fiddian-Qasmiyeh and Patricia Daley, 397–405. Abingdon: Routledge.

Ormond, Meghann and Neil Lunt. 2020. "Transnational medical travel: Patient mobility, shifting health system entitlements and attachments." *Journal of Ethnic and Migration Studies* 46 (20): 4179–92. doi:10.1080/1369183X.2019.1597465.

Pai, Sanjay A., and Sunil K. Pandya. 2010. "A revised Hippocratic oath for Indian medical students." *The National Medical Journal of India* 23 (6): 360.

Panda, Debashish. 2013. Working Group on Tertiary Care Institutions – 12th Plan, 29–30 November 2011. Planning Commission, Government of India.

Pandian, J. and S. Parman. 2004. The Making of Anthropology: The Semiotics of Self and Other in the Western Tradition. New Delhi: Vedams eBooks.

Parry, Jonathan. 1994. *Death in Banaras*. New York: Cambridge University Press.

Pellegrino, Edmund D. 1999. "The commodification of medical and health care: The moral consequences of a paradigm shift from a professional to a market ethic." *Journal of Medicine and Philosophy* 24 (3): 243–66.

Peters, Ellen, William Klein, Annette Kaufman, Louise Meilleur, and Anna Dixon. 2013. "More is not always better: Intuitions about effective public policy can lead to unintended consequences." *Social Issues and Policy Review* 7 (1): 114–48.

Planning Commission. 1950. *1st Five Year Plan*. New Delhi: Government of India.

Purohit, Brijesh C. 2001. "Private initiatives and policy options: Recent health system experience in India." *Health Policy and Planning* 16 (1): 87.

Qadeer, Imrana. 2000. "Health care systems in transition III. India, Part I. The Indian experience." *Journal of Public Health* 22 (1): 25–32.

Qadeer, Imrana. 2001. "Impact of structural adjustment programs of concepts in public health." In *Public Health and The Poverty of Reforms: The South Asian Predicament*, edited by Imrana Qadeer, Katsuri Sen and K. R. Nayar, 117–36. New Delhi, Thousand Oaks, London: Sage Publications.

Qadeer, Imrana. 2002. "Primary Health Care: From Adjustment to Reforms." In *Reforming India's Social Sector: Poverty, Nutrition, Health and Gender*, edited by K. Seeta Prabhu and R. Sudarshan, 221–31. New Delhi: Social Science Press.

Qadeer, Imrana, Katsuri Sen, and K. R. Nayar, eds. 2001. *Public Health and the Poverty of Reform: The South Asian Predicament*. New Delhi, Thousand Oaks, London: Sage Publications.

Qadeer, Imrana, and Sunita Reddy. 2013. "Medical tourism in India: Perceptions of physicians in tertiary care hospitals." *Philosophy, Ethics, and Humanities in Medicine* 8 (1): 20.

Rabinow, Paul. 2005. "Midst anthropology's problems." In *Global Assemblages: Technology, Politics, and Ethics as Anthropological Problems*, edited by Aiwa Ong and Stephen J. Collier, 40–54. Oxford, Malden & Carlton: Blackwell Publishing.

Radin, Margaret Jane. 2005. "Contested commodities." In *Rethinking Commodification: Cases and Readings in Law and Culture*, edited by Martha Ertman and Joan C. Williams, 81–95. New York: NYU Press.

Rajya Sabha Secretariat. 2012. Department Related Parliamentary Standing Committee on Health and Family Welfare: Fifty-ninth Report on the Functioning of the Central Drugs Standard Control Organisation. New Delhi: Parliament of India Rajya Sabha.

Raman, R., R. Rajalakshmi, J. Surya, R. Ramakrishnan, S. Sivaprasad, D. Conroy, J. Thethi, V. Mohan, and G. Netuveli. 2020. "Impact on health and provision of healthcare services during the COVID-19 lockdown in India: A multicentre cross-sectional study." *BMJ Open* 11: e043590. doi:10.1136/bmjopen-2020–043590.

Rao, Krishna D., Aarushi Bhatnagar, Peter Berman, I. Saran, and S. Raha. 2009. "India's health workforce: Size, composition and distribution." *India Health Beat. New Delhi: World Bank, New Delhi and Public Health Foundation of India* 1 (3): 1–4.

Rao, Mohan, Krishna D. Rao, A. K. Kumar, Mirai Chatterjee, and Thiagarajan Sundararaman. 2011. "Human resources for health in India." *The Lancet* 377 (9765): 587–98.

Rao, K. Sujatha, S. Selvaraju, Somil Nagpal, and S. Sakthivel. 2006. "Financing of health in India." In *Background Papers: Financing and Delivery of Health Care Services in India*. New Delhi: National Commission on Macroeconomics and Health, Ministry of Health and Family Welfare, Government of India.

Ravindran, G. D. 2008. "Medical ethics education in India." *Indian Journal of Medical Ethics* 5 (1): 18–19.

Reddy, Sunita, and Imrana Qadeer. 2010. "Medical tourism in India: Progress or predicament?." *Economic and Political Weekly* XLV (2): 69–75.

Riegel, Viviane. 2020. "The spaces of luxury in global cities: The consumption and appropriation of São Paulo's upscale malls by the elite and the poor." *HAU: Journal of Ethnographic Theory* 10 (1): 120–29.

Rekhi, D., and M. Akshatha. 2020. "Covid woes dent health tourism in South India; hospital revenues take a hit." *The Economic Times*. 6 October. Accessed 7 May 2021.

Riegel, Viviane. 2020. "The spaces of luxury in global cities: The consumption and appropriation of São Paulo's upscale malls by the elite and the poor." *HAU: Journal of Ethnographic Theory* 10 (1): 120–29.

Ritchie, Hannah. 2019. "Sanitation." Published online at OurWorldInData.org. https://ourworldindata.org/sanitation.

Roberts, Elizabeth, and Nancy Scheper-Hughes. 2011. "Introduction: Medical migrations." *Body & Society* 17 (2–3): 1–30.

Robinson, P., S. Heitmann, and P. Dieke. 2011. "Research themes in tourism: An introduction." In *Research Themes in Tourism*, edited by P. Robinson, S. Heitmann, and P. Dieke, xi–xvi. CAB International, Oxfordshire, UK.

Rolain, J. M., P. Parola, and G. Cornaglia. 2010. "New Delhi metallo-beta-lactamase (NDM-1): Towards a new pandemia?" *Clinical Microbiology and Infection* 16 (12): 1699–701.

Ross, G. F. 1994. *The Psychology of Tourism*. Hospitality Press Pty Ltd.

Roy, Ananya and Aihwa Ong, eds. 2011. *Worlding Cities: Asian Experiments and the Art of Being Global*. Oxford: Wiley Blackwell.

Roy, Ananya. 2011. "The blockade of the world-class city: Dialectical images of Indian urbanism." In *Worlding Cities: Asian Experiments and the Art of Being Global*, edited by Roy Ananya and Aihwa Ong, 259–78. Oxford: Wiley Blackwell.

Roy, Arundhati. 2021. "We are witnessing a crime against humanity: Arundhati Roy on India's Covid catastrophe." *The Guardian.* 29 April 2021. Accessed 19 June 2021. https://www.theguardian.com/news/2021/apr/28/crime-against-humanity -arundhati-roy-india-covid-catastrophe.

Roychowdhury, Viveka. 2009. "Reliance life sciences: A towering presence." *Express Pharma.* Accessed 18 December 2011. http://www.expresspharmaonline .com/20091115/expressbiotech11.shtml.

Rylko-Bauer, Barbara, and Paul Farmer. 2002. "Managed care or managed inequality? A call for critiques of market-based medicine." *Medical Anthropology Quarterly* 16 (4): 476.

Sachs, Wolfgang. 2002. "Fairness in a Fragile World: The Johannesburg Agenda." *Development* 45 (3): 12.

Saez, Lawrence, and Joy Yang. 2001. "The deregulation of state-owned enterprises in India and China." *Comparative Economic Studies* 43 (3): 69.

Salazar, Noel B. 2008. "Tourism imaginaries: A conceptual approach." *Annals of Tourism Research* 39 (2): 172–73.

Salazar, Noel B. 2012. "Tourism imaginaries: A conceptual approach." *Annals of Tourism Research* 39 (2): 863–82.

Salzar, Noel and Nelson H. H. Graburn, eds. 2014. *Tourism Imaginaries: Anthropological Approaches.* New York: Berghahn Books.

Salmon, J. Warren. 1984. "Organizing medical care for profit." In *Issues in the Political Economy of Health Care*, edited by John B. McKinlay, 143–86. Tavistock New York.

Scheper-Hughes, Nancy. 2000. "The global traffic in human organs." *Current Anthropology* 41 (2): 191–224.

Scheper-Hughes, Nancy. 2002a. "Bodies for sale – whole or in parts." In *Commodifying Bodies*, edited by Nancy Scheper-Hughes and Loic Wacquant, 1–8. London: Sage.

Scheper-Hughes, Nancy. 2002b. "The ends of the body: Commodity fetishism and the global raffic in organs." *SAIS Review* 22 (1): 61–80.

Scheper-Hughes, Nancy. 2003. "Keeping an eye on the global traffic in human organs." *The Lancet* 361 (9369): 1645–48.

Scheper-Hughes, Nancy. 2004. "Parts unknown undercover ethnography of the organs-trafficking underworld." *Ethnography* 5 (1): 29–73.

Scheper-Hughes, Nancy, and Loic Wacquant, eds. 2002. *Commodifying Bodies.* London: Sage.

Seifert-Granzin, Jörg, and D. Samuel Jesupatham. 1999. *Tourism at the Crossroads: Challenges to Developing Countries by the New World Trade Order.* Vol. 96. Frankfurt: Equations, Tourism Watch (ZEB).

Selvaraj S., H. H. Farooqui, and A. Karan. 2018. "Quantifying the financial burden of households' out-of-pocket payments on medicines in India: A repeated cross-sectional analysis of National Sample Survey data, 1994–2014." *BMJ Open.* 8 (5): e018020.

Sen, Amartya. 2001. *Development as Freedom.* Oxford, UK: Oxford Paperbacks.

Sen, Amartya, and Jean Dreze. 1999. The Amartya Sen and Jean Drèze Omnibus: (comprising) Poverty and Famines; Hunger and Public Action; and India:

Economic Development and Social Opportunity. New Delhi: Oxford University Press.

Sen, Siddhartha. 1992. "Non-profit organisations in India: Historical development and common patterns." *Voluntas: International Journal of Voluntary and Nonprofit Organizations* 3 (2): 175–93.

Sengupta, Amit and Samiran Nundy. 2005. "The private health sector in India." *BMJ* 331 (7526): 1157–58.

Shekhar, Mayank. 2011. "The Mumbai of clichés." *Hindustan Times*. Accessed 21 January 2021. https://www.hindustantimes.com/entertainment/the-mumbai-of-cliches/story-0VVtbNB5xvdbpUTpq6BFiO.html.

Singer, Merrill. 2009. "Pathogens gone wild? Medical anthropology and the "swine flu" pandemic." *Medical Anthropology* 28 (3): 199–206.

Singer, Merrill. 2014. "Following the turkey tails: Neoliberal globalization and the political ecology of health." *Journal of Political Ecology* 21: 436–51.

Singer, Merrill, and Arachu Castro. 2004. Unhealthy Health Policy: A Critical Anthropological Examination. Rowman Altamira.

Singer, Merrill, and Hans Baer. 1995. "Critical medical anthropology." *Anthropological Quarterly* 11: 224–45.

Singer, Merrill, and Hans Baer. 2012. *Introducing Medical Anthropology: A Discipline in Action.* Plymouth, UK: AltaMira Press. Accessed 22 March 2016.

Singh, L. 2014. "An evaluation of medical tourism in India." *African Journal of Hospitality, Tourism and Leisure* 3 (1): 1–11.

Singh, Nancy. 2005. "Branding is empowerment of the Indian healthcare consumer." *Express Healthcare Management.* Accessed 29 March 2012. http://www.express healthcaremgmt.com/20050131/branding02.shtml.

Singh, Nancy. 2008. "Corporate governance on healthcare's platter." *Express Healthcare.* Accessed 23 September 2009. http://archivehealthcare.financialexpress.com/200802/coverstory01.shtml.

Singh, R. and P. Rana. 2001. "The future of heritage tourism in Varanasi: Scenario, prospects and perspectives." *National Geographical Journal of India* 47: 201–18.

Siyam, Amani, and Mario Roberto Dal Poz, eds. 2014. *Migration of Health Workers: WHO Code of Practice and the Global Economic Crisis.* Geneva: World Health Organization.

Smith-Morris, Carolyn, and Lenore Manderson. 2010. "The Baggage of Health Travelers." *Medical Anthropology* 29 (4): 331–35.

Smith-Oka, Vania. 2009. "Unintended consequences: Exploring the tensions between development programs and indigenous women in Mexico in the context of reproductive health." *Social Science & Medicine* 68 (11): 2069–77.

Snyder, Jeremy, Tsogtbaatar Byambaa, Rory Johnston, Valorie A. Crooks, Craig Janes, and Melanie Ewan. 2015. "Outbound medical tourism from Mongolia: A qualitative examination of proposed domestic health system and policy responses to this trend." *BMC Health Services Research* 15 (1): 1.

Snyder, Jeremy, Valorie A. Crooks, Leigh Turner, and Rory Johnston. 2013. "Understanding the impacts of medical tourism on health human resources in Barbados: A prospective, qualitative study of stakeholder perceptions." *International Journal for Equity in Health* 12 (2). https://doi.org/10.1186/1475-9276-12-2.

Sobo, Elisa J. 2011. "Medical anthropology in disciplinary context: Definitional struggles and key debates (or answering the Cri du Coeur)." In *A Companion to Medical Anthropology*, edited by M. Singer and P. I. Erickson, 9–28. West Sussex, UK: John Wiley & Sons Ltd.

Song, Priscilla. 2010. "Biotech pilgrims and the transnational quest for stem cell cures." *Medical Anthropology* 29 (4): 384–402.

Solomon, Harris. 2011. "Affective journeys: The emotional structuring of medical tourism in India." *Anthropology and Medicine* 18 (1): 105–18.

Sookrajh, Reshma. 2011. "Volunatarism as civic action: Reflections from religious Hindu organizations in South Africa." *Man In India* 91 (1): 73–92.

Speier, Amy. 2016. Fertility Holidays: IVF Tourism and the Reproduction of Whiteness. New York: NYU Press, 2016.

Stiglitz, J. E. 2002. *Globalization and its Discontents*. New York: Norton & Company.

Stiglitz, J. E. 2008. "Capital market liberalization, globalization, and the IMF." In *Capital Market Liberalization and Development*, edited by Jose Antonio Ocampo and Joseph Stiglitz, 76–100. New York: Oxford University Press.

Stiglitz, J. E. 2012. *The Price of Inequality*. London: Penguin Books Ltd.

"Stricter visa rules driving away medical tourism from India." 2013. *The Economic Times,* August 19. Accessed 18 August 2013. https://economictimes.indiatimes .com/nri/visa-and-immigration/stricter-visa-rules-driving-away-medical-tourism -from-india/articleshow/21836093.cms.

Stuckler, David, and Sanjay Basu. 2009. "The International Monetary Fund's effects on global health: Before and after the 2008 financial crisis." *International Journal of Health Services* 39 (4): 771–81.

Taylor, Sebastian. 2018. "'Global health': Meaning what?" *BMJ Global Health* 2018 (3): e000843.

Teh, Ivy. 2007. "Healthcare tourism in Thailand: Pain ahead?" *Asia Pacific Biotech News (APBN)* 11 (8): 493–97.

Telej, E. and J. R. Gamble. 2019. "Yoga wellness tourism: A study of marketing strategies in India." *Journal of Consumer Marketing* 36 (6): 794–805.

Terry, Nicolas. 2007. "Under-regulated healthcare phenomena in a flat world: Medical tourism and outsourcing." *Western New England Law Review* 29. Accessed 17 July 2012.

Thomas, George, and Joe Varghese. 2010. "Gifts to doctors, scientific information and the credibility gap in the Medical Council of India." *Indian Journal of Medical Ethics* 7 (2): 68–69.

Transparency International. 2006. *Global Corruption Report 2006*. London; Ann Arbor, MI: Pluto Press/Transparency International.

Turner, Leigh. 2007. "First world health care at third world prices: Globalization, bioethics and medical tourism." *BioSocieties* 2: 303–25.

UNESCO Institute for Statistics. 2014. *Global flow of tertiary-level students*, accessed 25 November 2015, http://www.uis.unesco.org/Education/Pages/interna-tional-student-flow-viz.aspx.

United Nations. 1948. "Universal declaration of human rights." In *General Assembly res 217A (III)*.

United Nations. 2010. *World Urbanization Prospects: The 2009 Revision*. New York: United Nations Department of Economic and Social Affairs.

United Nations. 2018. *The World's Cities in 2018—Data Booklet*. New York: Department of Economic and Social Affairs. Accessed 14 June 2021. https://www .un.org/en/events/citiesday/assets/pdf/the_worlds_cities_in_2018_data_booklet .pdf.

United Nations Development Program. 2005. "Human development report 2005: International cooperation at a crossroads: Aid, trad and security in an unequal world." In *Human Development Report 2005*. New York: UNDP.

United Nations Development Program. 2009. Human Development Report 2009: Overcoming Barriers: Human Mobility and Development. New York: Palgrave Macmillan.

United Nations Development Program. 2010. *Mumbai Human Development Report 2009*. New Delhi: Oxford University Press.

United Nations Development Program. 2014. Human Development Report 2014: Sustaining Human Progress: Reducing Vulnerabilities and Building Resilience. New York: UNDP.

United Nations Economic and Social Council. 2000. "The right to the highest attainable standard of health." Committee on Economic, Social and Cultural Rights, Geneva, 25 April–12 May 2000.

United Nations Habitat. 2003. Understanding Slums: Case Study for the Global Report on Human Settlements. London: Earthscan.

United Nations Habitat. 2015. "Housing and slum upgrading." United Nations. Accessed 1 September 2015. http://unhabitat.org/urban-themes/housing-slum -upgrading/.

United Nations Habitat. 2018. *SDG Indicator 11.1.1 Training Module: Adequate Housing and Slum Upgrading*. Nairobi: United Nations Human Settlement Programme (UN-Habitat).

United Nations High Commissioner on Human Rights, Economic, Social, and Cultural Rights. 2004. "Special rapporteurs on rights to health and education present findings to commission." *Press Document*.

United Nations Statistics Division. 2015. "Births attended by skilled health personnel, percentage." In *Millenium Development Goals Database*. New York: United Nations.

United Nations World Tourism Organisation. 2020. *UNWTO World Tourism Barometer* (Vol. 18, Issue 2, May 2020). Madrid, Spain: UNWTO.

United States Congress. 2006. Special Committee on Aging. The Globalization of Health Care: Can Medical Tourism Reduce Health Care Costs? Second. June 27.

Van Der Geest, Sjaak, and Kaja Finkler. 2004. "Hospital ethnography: Introduction." *Social Science & Medicine* 59: 1995–2001.

Van Doorslaer, Eddy, Owen O'Donnell, Ravi P Rannan-Eliya, Aparnaa Somanathan, Shiva Raj Adhikari, Charu C Garg, Deni Harbianto, Alejandro N. Herrin, Mohammed Nazmul Huq, and Shamsia Ibragimova. 2006. "Effect of payments for health care on poverty estimates in 11 countries in Asia: an analysis of household survey data." *The lancet* 368 (9544): 1357–64.

"Varun Dhawan receive first dose of Covid-19 vaccine, thanks the 'wonderful doctors." 2021. *Hindustan Times.* 19 June. Accessed 20 June 2021. https://www .hindustantimes.com/entertainment/bollywood/varun-dhawan-receives-first-dose -of-covid-19-vaccine-thanks-the-wonderful-doctors-see-here-101624096437994 .html.

Vequist, D. G., M. Guiry, and B. Ipock. 2012. "Controversies in medical tourism." In *Controversies in Tourism,* edited by Omar Moufakkir and Peter M. Burns. Oxfordshire, UK: CABI.

Viladrich, A., and R. Baron-Faust. 2014. "Medical tourism in tango paradise: The internet branding of cosmetic surgery in Argentina." *Annals of Tourism Research* 45: 116–31. doi:10.1016/j.annals.2013.12.007.

Wagstaff, Adam. 2002. "Inequalities in health in developing countries: Swimming against the tide?" In *Policy Research Working Paper 2795.* Washington, D.C.: The World Bank.

Waitzkin, Howard, ed. 2000. *The Second Sickness: Contradictions of Capitalist Health Care.* Revised and Updated ed. Oxford: Rowman & Littlefield Publishers.

Waldrop, Annie. 2004. "Gating and class relations: The case of a New Delhi "colony"." *City & Society* 16 (2): 93–116.

Wallerstein, Immanuel. 1974a. The Modern World System, Volume 1: Capitalist Agriculture and the Origins of the European World-Economy in the Sixteenth Century. New York, London: Academic Press.

Wallerstein, Immanuel. 1974b. "The rise and future demise of the world capitalist system: Concepts for comparative analysis." *Comparative Studies in Society and History* 16 (4): 387–415.

Wallerstein, Immanuel. 1979. *The Capitalist World-Economy: Essays.* New York: Cambridge University Press.

Walton-Roberts, Margaret. 2015. "International migration of health professionals and the marketization and privatization of health education in India: From push–pull to global political economy." *Social Science & Medicine* 124: 374–82.

Whiteford, Linda M. 2000. "Local identify, globalization and health in Cuba and the Dominican Republic." In *Global Health Policy, Local Realities: The Fallacy of a Level-playing Field,* edited by Linda M. Whiteford and Lenore Manderson, 57–78. Boulder, CO: Lynne Rienner Publishers.

Whitehead, Margaret. 1991. "The concepts and principles of equity and health." *Health Promotion International* 6 (3): 217–28.

Whittaker, Andrea. 2007. "Medical tourism in Asia." In *Melbourne University Up Close.* Australia: The University of Melbourne.

Whittaker, Andrea. 2008. "Pleasure and pain: Medical travel in Asia." *Global Public Health* 3 (3): 271–90.

Whittaker, Andrea, Lenore Manderson, and Elizabeth Cartwright. 2010. "Patients without Borders: Understanding medical travel." *Medical Anthropology* 29 (4): 336–43.

Whittaker, Andrea, and Amy Speier. 2010. "Cycling overseas: Care, commodification, and stratification in cross-border reproductive travel." *Medical Anthropology: Cross-Cultural Studies in Health and Illness* 29 (4): 363–83.

Whittaker, Andrea, and Chee Heng Leng. "'Flexible bio-citizenship' and international medical travel: Transnational mobilities for care in Asia." *International Sociology* 31 (3): 286–304.

Winter, Tim, Peggy Teo, and T. C. Chang. 2009. *Asia on Tour: Exploring the Rise of Asian Tourism*. New York: Routledge.

World Bank. 1987. "Financing health services in developing countries: An agenda for reform." In *World Bank Strategy Paper*. New York: Oxford University Press.

World Bank. 1993. *World Development Report: Investing in Health*. New York: Oxford University Press.

World Bank. 1996. "Structural adjustment in India." In *OED Evaluation Report Precis*. Geneva: World Bank.

World Bank. 2009. *Reshaping Economic Geography*. Washington DC: World Bank.

World Bank. 2011. Perspectives on Poverty in India: Stylized Facts from Survey Data. Washington, DC: World Bank.

World Bank. 2014. *World Development Indicators*. Washington, DC: The World Bank.

World Bank. 2020. *Prevalence of Undernourishment (% of Population)*. Washington, D.C.: The World Bank. Accessed 3 May 2021. https://data.worldbank.org/indicator /SN.ITK.DEFC.ZS.

World Bank. 2021a. *World Bank Open Data: India*. Washington: World Bank. Accessed 9 Jun 2021. https://data.worldbank.org/country/india?view=chart.

World Bank. 2021b. *Domestic General Government Health Expenditure*. Washington: World Bank. Accessed 9 June 2021. https://data.worldbank.org/indicator/SH.XPD .GHED.CH.ZS.

World Bank. 2021c. *World Bank Group Finances*. Washington, D.C.: The World Bank. Accessed 4 June 2021. https://finances.worldbank.org/Loans-and-Credits/ total-loan-of-india-that-pay/7tnf-rf6t/data.

World Health Organization. 2001. *Country Health Profile*. India: WHO.

World Health Organization. 2009. *World Health Statistics 2009*. Geneva: WHO.

World Health Organization. 2010. *WHO Global Code of Practice on the International Recruitment of Health Personnel*. Geneva: WHA63.16, Sixty-third World Health Assembly.

World Health Organization. 2014a. "Global health observatory data repository." In *Density by Country: Data by Country*. Geneva: WHO.

World Health Organization. 2014b. *Global Tuberculosis Report 2014*. Geneva: WHO.

World Health Organization. 2014c. *World Health Statistics 2014*. Geneva: WHO.

World Health Organization. 2015a. "Health systems strengthening glossary." WHO. Accessed 8 October 2015. http://www.who.int/healthsystems/hss_glossary/en/ index5.html.

World Health Organization. 2015b. *World Health Statistics 2015*. Geneva, Switzerland: WHO.

World Health Organization. 2020a. "Countries are spending more on health, but people are still paying too much out of their own pockets." *News*. Geneva, Switzerland: WHO. Accessed 13 June 2021. https://www.who.int/news/item/20

-02-2019-countries-are-spending-more-on-health-but-people-are-still-paying-too -much-out-of-their-own-pockets.

World Health Organisation. 2020b. *World Health Statistics 2021: Monitoring Health for the SDGs*. Geneva: WHO. Accessed 31 May 2021. https://cdn.who.int/media/ docs/default-source/gho-documents/world-health-statistic-reports/2021/whs-2021 _20may.pdf?sfvrsn=55c7c6f2_8.

World Health Organization. 2020c. *Decade for Health Workforce Strengthening in SEAR 2015–2024, Mid-Term Review Of Progress*. Geneva: World Health Organization. Accessed 20 June 2021. https://apps.who.int/iris/handle/10665 /333611.

World Health Organization. 2021. *Global Health Estimates: Life Expectancy and Leading Causes of Death and Disability*. Geneva, Switzerland: WHO. Accessed 9 June 2021. https://www.who.int/data/gho/data/themes/mortality-and-global-health -estimates.

World Trade Organization. 1998. Health and Social Services: Background Note by the Secretariat, S/C/W/50, 98-3558. New York: WTO.

World Trade Organization. 2001. "Communication from Cuba, Dominican Republic, Haiti, India, Kenya, Pakistan, Peru, Uganda, Venezuela and Zimbabwe." Accessed 21 September 2009. http://www.wto.org/english/tratop_e/serv_e/s_propnewnegs _e.htm.

Wright Jr, Theodore P. 1975. "Competitive Modernization within the Daudi Bohra Sect of Muslims and its Significance for Indian Political Development." In *Competition and modernization in South Asia*, edited by Helen E. Ulrich, 151–178.

Xu, K., A. Soucat, J. Kutzin, C. Brindley, N. Vande Maele, H. Tour, M. Aranguren Garcia, D. Li, H. Barroy, G. Flores, T. Roubal, C. Indikadahena, V. Cherilova, and A. Siroka. 2018. "Public spending on health: A closer look at global trends." *HF Working Paper*. 18.3. Geneva: World Health Organization.

Yadav, Kapil, S. V. Nikhil, and Chandrakant S. Pandav. 2011. "Urbanization and health challenges: Need to fast track launch of the National Urban Health Mission." *Indian Journal of Community Medicine: Official Publication of Indian Association of Preventive & Social Medicine* 36 (1): 3.

Yamashita, S., A. K. H. Din, and J. S. Eades. 1997. *Tourism and Cultural Development in Asia and Oceania*. Selangor, Malaysia: Penerbit Universiti Kebangsaan Malaysia.

Yamey, G. 2001. "World Bank funds private hospital in India." *BMJ: British Medical Journal* 322 (7281): 257.

Yesudian, C. A. K. 1999. "Pattern of utilisation of health services: Policy implica- tions." *Economic and Political Weekly* 34 (5): 300–4.

Young, Aaron, Humayun J. Chaudhry, Janelle Rhyne, and Michael Dugan. 2011. "A census of actively licensed physicians in the United States, 2010." *Journal of Medical Regulation* 96 (4): 10–20.

Index

Page numbers in *italics* refer to Figures and Tables.

About the Author

Kristen Smith is a senior research fellow based at the University of Melbourne, Australia. Trained as a medical anthropologist, her research interests include medical tourism in India, as well as globalization, political economy, development, mobility, health equity, and Indigenous studies.

www.ingramcontent.com/pod-product-compliance
Lightning Source LLC
Chambersburg PA
CBHW022312280326
41932CB00010B/1079